*Jesus asked the lame man by the pool of Bethesda,
"Wilt thou be made whole?"*

Whole-Person Medicine

An International Symposium

*edited by David F. Allen, Lewis Penhall Bird
and Robert L. Herrmann*

*InterVarsity Press
Downers Grove
Illinois 60515*

InterVarsity Press is the book-publishing division of Inter-Varsity Christian Fellowship, a student movement active on campus at hundreds of universities, colleges and schools of nursing. For information about local and regional activities, write IVCF, 233 Langdon St., Madison, WI 53703.

Distributed in Canada through InterVarsity Press, 1875 Leslie St., Unit 10, Don Mills, Ontario M3B 2M5, Canada.

"A Clinical View of the Gospel" © 1980 by Bruce Larson and used by permission of the author.

All Scripture quotations, unless otherwise indicated, are from the Revised Standard Version of the Bible, copyrighted 1946, 1952, © 1971, 1973, and are used by permission.

ISBN 0-87784-815-7

Printed in the United States of America

Library of Congress Cataloging in Publication Data
Main entry under title:
Whole-person medicine.
    Papers presented in Feb. 1979 at an international symposium held at the Oral Roberts University School of Medicine in Tulsa, Oklahoma.
    Includes bibliographical references.
    1. Medicine–Philosophy–Congresses. 2. Medicine and Christianity–Congresses. 3. Holistic medicine–Congresses. 4. Physician and patient–Congresses. 5. Medical ethics–Congresses. I. Allen, David Franklyn. II. Bird, Lewis P. III. Herrmann, Robert L., 1928-   IV. Oral Roberts University. School of Medicine. [DNLM: 1. Holistic health–Congresses. 2. Religion and medicine–Congresses. W61 I625w 1979]
R723.W47   610.69'6   79-2807
ISBN 0-87784-815-7

17   16   15   14   13   12   11   10   9   8   7   6   5   4   3   2   1
94   93   92   91   90   89   88   87   86   85   84   83   82   81   80

Introduction

In our fractured world, deceit, dysfunction and distance separate one individual from another. The promise of new
beginnings, new birth and restoration to wholeness touches
the spirit of each of us. In their quest for wholeness, patients
(or clients) turn to the health-care delivery system and to the
helping professions. Many consumers and clinicians want to
move beyond present practice to approaches designed to restore wholeness. Are the healing arts prepared to meet such
expectations?

Although "holistic" or "wholistic" or "whole-person" medicine often receives affirmation today, the basis for that affirmation varies widely. In some instances its roots are in
magic and mysticism, blending the cultic with the unconventional in a way that defies scientific medicine and deifies alien
forces. A recent medical editorial warns of "the irrational
side of the holistic movement, with its mystical cults and all the
paraphernalia of sectarianism."[1] Philosophical as well as
scientific discernment is needed; clinical pitfalls and fads must
be avoided and the patient's (and professional's) personhood
must not be violated.

The papers in this volume were presented in February

1979 at an international symposium held at the Oral Roberts University School of Medicine in Tulsa, Oklahoma. The purpose of the symposium was to define and examine the theme, "Whole-Person Medicine," and to establish goals as a foundation for related educational programs. The shared Christian faith of the conferees enabled emphasis to be placed on the transcendent value of every individual, the divinely bestowed character of human beings and the grace available in health and illness. Continually underscored was a need to integrate modern scientific medicine and clinical excellence with sensitivity to the spiritual dimensions of the patient.[2]

Biblically speaking, *health* and *salvation* share the same linguistic roots. Hence a lively biblical faith can meet disease, dysfunction and distance with a reconciling, restorative regimen rooted in profound awareness of the interworkings of body and spirit. Guilt, alienation, low self-esteem and lack of self-discipline contribute to personal distress. Physicians with a Christian faith acknowledge the remarkable healing of human dis-ease that can occur when the divine touches the human. For Christians, human wholeness finds its ultimate example in the life and ministry of Jesus Christ. Countless patients have begun a pilgrimage to personal wholeness when Christ's presence has transformed both their illness and their alienation. In such a personal encounter, grace and forgiveness offer the promise of a "new becoming" (2 Cor. 5:17).

For the discovery (or perhaps recovery) of a conceptual basis for wholistic medicine,[3] perspectives can be gathered from a biblical faith that can provide a theological foundation on which such a health-care system may be established. The Judeo-Christian tradition recognizes a sense of disintegration and alienation introduced into our cosmos with the intrusion of evil and the Fall of man (Gen. 3). Biblical faith does not portray a false optimism about any inherent capability of individuals to resolve their dilemmas on a purely human level. Rather, it first paints a realistic panorama of human beings estranged at all levels of existence. Incarnational love then seeks to bring order out of chaos, wholeness from brokenness, and healing where dysfunction has destroyed health.

Wholeness in biblical faith can be defined in several ways. In such motifs, clinicians may discover compelling insights for the treatment of the patient, insights that will more fully enhance human dignity and alleviate human suffering.

Theological Themes

First, Holy Scripture depicts an *integrated, pristine creation,* devoid of dysfunction or estrangement. Scripture reveals that "God saw everything that he had made, and behold, it was very good" (Gen. 1:31). From the almighty and loving Spirit behind the universe came a new creation of harmony and balance. No record of human disease, alienation, perversity or deviancy marred that Edenic paradise.

The Westminster Larger Catechism describes that original estate:

> The providence of God toward man in the estate in which he was created was the placing him in paradise, appointing him to dress it, giving him liberty to eat of the fruit of the earth; putting the creatures under his dominion, and ordaining marriage for his help; affording him communion with himself; instituting the sabbath; entering into a covenant of life with him, upon condition of personal, perfect, and perpetual obedience, of which the tree of life was a pledge; and forbidding [him] to eat of the tree of the knowledge of good and evil, upon the pain of death.

At the outset of their pilgrimage, human beings were placed in an environment of innocence, free of malevolent forces and without shame of estrangement, in perfect union with their Creator. Part of the current quest for human wholeness surely derives from a desire to regain what might have been. Creation culminated in the establishment on earth of God's vice regents created in the divine image as male and female humans, having dominion over living things.

Integrated human personhood is a second motif that can illumine and govern whole-person health care. Centuries of debate over the biblical words for body, soul, spirit, heart, will, bowels and so on produced theories of a two-part (dichotomous) or three-part (trichotomous) human being, but twentieth-century theologians have come to acknowledge the essential wholism of individual human life.

In brief, examination of the Hebrew words *nephesh, ruach* and *leb* or *lebab* ("living soul," "spirit" and "heart") discloses a wide range of often overlapping aspects of human nature. Any clear compartmentalization of either form or function is precluded. With reference to *nephesh,* one scholar speaks of a "chaos of meanings" that the term engenders.[4] It may stand for breath, the power of life, life itself, the seat of desire, the seat of physical affections, a person, a man or someone. *Ruach* can speak of the energy of life, wind, the Spirit of God and human life itself; its range is not exclusive of *nephesh* at all. And *leb* usually means "the total orientation, direction, concentration of man, his depth dimension, from which his full human existence is directed and formed."[5]

New Testament references have often been appealed to by those seeking a basis for either human dichotomy or trichotomy. Hebrews 4:12 speaks of the "piercing to the division of soul and spirit" and 1 Thessalonians 5:23 considers the preservation of "spirit and soul and body." The *locus classicus* of a two-part nature (body and soul), "Then the LORD God formed man of dust from the ground, and breathed into his nostrils the breath of life; and man became a living being" (Gen. 2:7), is echoed in 1 Corinthians 15:45: "The first man Adam became a living being; the last Adam became a life-giving spirit." But then Matthew 22:37 speaks of loving the Lord your God "with all your heart, and with all your soul, and with all your mind." Mark 12:30 adds to these "and with all your strength."

Aware that in biblical anthropology diverse terms may describe various functions of an intact human being, many distinguished theologians have now acknowledged that "Hebraic holism" does justice to the biblical record more completely than either of the older explanations.[6] Biblical anthropology underscores the interrelatedness of all elements of human nature and their common expression in the experience of any solitary individual at a given place in time. Modern medical awareness which recognizes the interplay between one's physical state and one's inner being thus finds ample support in Scripture.

A third motif confronts us all, however, namely, our *fragmented human experience*. Everyone experiences personal, social, environmental or metaphysical dysfunction at one time or another. Although we may perceive a wholistic interrelatedness of our personal lives, fractures in body and spirit are not foreign to any of us. Disorientation in society, dislocations in the environment and alienation from any governing metaphysical meaning of life afflict the human spirit and create a deep longing for reconciliation. Many modern writers portray such longing.

The ministry of Jesus found remarkable cohesion in response to this brokenness. " 'But that you may know that the Son of man has authority on earth to forgive sins'—he said to the paralytic—'I say to you, rise, take up your pallet and go home' " (Mk. 2:10-11). Jesus' remarkable ability touched both the spirit and the body of the sufferer. The man left that encounter restored in more dimensions of his being than had been anticipated by skeptical onlookers.

The apostle Paul analyzed the inner turmoil of the fallen human condition: "For I do not do the good I want, but the evil I do not want is what I do" (Rom. 7:19). Whether one is overweight, abusive of a spouse, without meaning in life, bored, addicted, undisciplined, unable to handle stress, overworked, oppressed or neurotic, our common human estrangement is daily in evidence.

Channeling of the Spirit of Christ through his servants in the healing professions makes possible the healing or restoration of these various fractures at deeper levels than would be possible in conventional medicine. The hospice movement and Alcoholics Anonymous have been two successful medical experiments where wholistic treatment-plans have included both family members and the divine presence. They have ministered to the various levels of patient need in a thorough manner. The former movement has supported the dying patient and, unlike other therapy regimens, has consistently controlled pain, maintained an unclouded patient sensorium and incorporated family members in the final months of a loved one's life. The latter group has seen many remarkable recoveries that have withstood the test of time.

Those examples of wholistic treatment suggest the untapped power within family systems, meaningful value systems and medical care that results from practitioners as whole persons responding to patients as whole persons. The witness of transformed marriages, reconciled families, reclaimed jobs, recovered health and restored spirits underscores how dramatically whole-person care can transcend routinized patient-professional interactons.

A fourth relevant theological motif is the *wholistic eschatological restoration* envisioned in Scripture as a capstone to history. The suffering of all creation "waits with eager longing ... because the creation itself will be set free from its bondage to decay. . . . The whole creation has been groaning in travail together until now; and not only the creation, but we ourselves, who have the first fruits of the Spirit" (Rom. 8:19, 21-23). Whether the view of liberation is Paul's or the prophet Isaiah's—"The wolf shall dwell with the lamb, and the leopard shall lie down with the kid, and the calf and the lion and the fatling together, and a little child shall lead them" (Is. 11:6; 65:25)—a new earth is envisioned as a place where original wholeness, integration, and harmonious (holy) living will be restored.

From memories of a pristine integration of life before the ruinations of evil, to a future where order is restored and justice prevails, part of the Christian's hope is to see creation in balance and the whole scheme of life devoid of dysfunction, disease and death. The Incarnation as a historical event offers a foresight and hope and a perspective that encourages the present appropriation of divine grace as a forerunner of future wholeness. With the knowledge that history is moving toward perfection in the reign of Christ, movement toward personal wholeness now anticipates ultimate triumph.

Linguistic Themes
At least two literary motifs offer additional perspectives on

whole-person medicine from Christian belief. First, Greek understanding of *health* and *salvation* reveals a legitimate relationship. That family of word-stems suggests restoration, relief and reconciliation.

The Greek word for "savior," *soter*, applied in the New Testament uniquely to Jesus of Nazareth (Jn. 4:42; Acts 13: 23; Phil. 3:20; 1 Tim. 1:1; 2 Pet. 1:1), had a broad historical precedent. It could be applied to philosophers (who might save one from meaninglessness in life), statesmen (who might save one from social and political crises) and physicians (who might save one from the processes of disease). Jesus as Savior delivered people from both their sins and their diseases. Noteworthy was his reference point in Isaiah's prophecy: " 'The Spirit of the Lord is upon me, because he has anointed me to preach good news to the poor. He has sent me to proclaim release to the captives, and recovering of sight to the blind, to set at liberty those who are oppressed, to proclaim the acceptable year of the Lord.' And he closed the book, and gave it back to the attendant, and sat down [and said], 'Today this scripture has been fulfilled in your hearing' " (Lk. 4:18-21; Is. 61:1-2). The prophet had envisioned a day when Messiah would minister to the various needs of people. Jesus proclaimed the day when such a total ministry was in practice.

In Hellenistic literature the word "to save," *sozo*, was used of being saved from serious peril, from shipwreck, from the dangers of war, from judicial condemnation, from the risks of sailing and from illness. It could also refer to being pardoned as a lawbreaker. In medical parlance, it would mean to be cured, to stay in good health or to preserve one's inner or emotional equilibrium. As a term rich with medical, social and religious meanings, its application to the work of Jesus carried a powerful message about a diverse ministry which embodied many of those options.

The Gospels used the word to speak of Jesus' mission; for example, in Matthew 1:21, "For he will save his people from their sins."

In spiritual redemption, it is used in reference to being made whole: "For she said within herself, If I may but touch his garment, I shall be whole" (Mt. 9:21 KJV); "Thy faith hath made thee whole" (Mt. 9:22 KJV); "And as many as touched him were made whole" (Mk. 6:56 KJV).

A word rich in heritage became capable of multiple meanings in the ministry of Jesus. The author of Hebrews may have had in mind "such a great salvation" (Heb. 2:2) in recounting the signs, wonders, miracles and gifts vested in that remarkable Man. Medical mission enterprises have long recognized the interrelationship between health and salvation. Perhaps modern clinical medicine in metropolitan or suburban offices should adopt a medical model that Christian physicians practice in third-world countries (where spiritual oppression has at times been more obvious).

A second word rich in both medical and spiritual meaning is the Hebrew word for peace, *shalom*. The Hebrew *shalem*, which means "healthy" or "whole," is a cognate of *shalom*. Together they suggest a total well-being, a wholeness of personhood. When the various human physiological systems in dynamic equilibrium are perceived to be "at peace," health ensues. As peace permeates inner chaos, social conflict, environmental disequilibrium and metaphysical estrangement, God's Spirit provides his *shalom* to persons created in his image and who thus are restless for peace. The Mosaic benediction blends health with wholeness. "The LORD bless you and keep you: The LORD make his face to shine upon you, and be gracious to you: The LORD lift up his countenance upon you, and give you peace [*shalom*]" (Num. 6:24-26). The poetic parallelism found in the psalms flows through all of Psalm 29, culminating in a blend of health and total well-being: "May the LORD give strength to his people! May the LORD bless his people with peace!" (Ps. 29:11).

Lamenting over the passage of time, the writer of Ecclesiastes provided a commentary on "a time for war, and a time for [*shalom*]," "a time to break down, and a time to build up" and "a time to kill, and a time to heal" (Eccles. 3:3). The prophet Jeremiah described acute suffering amid the absence of health or well-being: "We have heard a cry of panic, of terror, and no peace" (Jer. 30:5). In contrast, the prophet Isaiah spoke of God's loyal covenant of peace in the midst of incredible suffering: "For the mountains may depart and the hills be removed, but my steadfast love shall not depart from you, and my covenant of peace shall not be removed, says the LORD, who has compassion on you" (Is. 54:10).

With *shalom* comes tranquillity, equilibrium, perspective, health, peace, even when surrounded by turmoil. The Hebrew blessing speaks of a richness of life transcending bodily health or emotional stability; the depths of one's whole being are touched by God's permanent, personal peace. Perhaps Old Testament scholar J. Barton Payne best captured the special quality of God's *shalom:* "this term carries with it, positively, the rich implications of soundness and wholeness, of that full integration of life which becomes possible only for those who live in tune with the One who is the Master of all that a [person] may encounter."[7]

Cosmic wholeness, part of our origin and heritage, is the reference point toward which all creation moves as the "day of the Lord" approaches. Though we are unified in being, our broken-ness is evident in disease. Our return to health, healed relationships, and recovery of meaning, as well as our efforts at ecological balance, indicate a longing for a larger healing, a richer wholeness for life.

Symposium Sponsors

With the biblical challenge to wholeness in mind, the International Symposium on Whole-Person Medicine was organized by the Christian Medical Society and the Oral Roberts University Medical School.

Christian Medical Society. The Christian Medical Society, an international group of physicians, dentists and students preparing for these professions, is deeply committed to the teachings and lordship of Jesus Christ. CMS seeks to integrate biblical principles and the practice of medicine through conferences, symposia, retreats, a journal and social action programs. Emphasis is placed on mature spirituality and excellence in medical practice, on the dignity and human rights of all persons. Medical students are encouraged to examine their belief-structures as those relate to their development in the field of medicine. Dedicated to serving Jesus Christ in and through the medical and dental professions, CMS seeks to help men and women become whole in the confidence that this twentieth-century world belongs to God, and that Christ is its hope.

Oral Roberts University. Oral Roberts University's interest in whole-person medicine stems from its original commitment, over fifteen years ago, to educate the whole person: body, mind and spirit. Oral Roberts's ministry of healing, a forerunner and now companion of the university, has been strengthened and broadened through the establishment of professional schools in medicine, dentistry, nursing and law. Those programs complement already existing graduate programs in theology and business. Accreditation for medicine and dentistry was granted in 1978; law was scheduled to begin in the fall of 1979. When graduate nursing joins the six-year-old undergraduate nursing program, the complete group will all be housed in one large graduate center.

Locating the six professional schools under one roof encourages an integrative program. Students are exposed to a multidisciplinary approach to health care (a "cross-pollination"). The four major categories—business, law, health care and theology—pertain to major life experiences of every individual. Experiences in buying and selling, in abiding by the law, in dealing with illness and in resolving one's own value system in light of personal faith in God—these are the "stuff of life." Physicians are trained to minister to their patients with sensitivity to all individual needs. That in no way diminishes the technical aspects of medical education; rather it enlarges the student's awareness of all aspects of human health and personal need.

Physicians who are both technically competent and humanly sensitive are as ready to refer patients to a minister, financial adviser or other counselor when appropriate, as to a specialist in another medical field. Applying the whole-person approach to health-care education and patient care, Oral Roberts has formed "healing teams." Teams of health-care professionals, ministers, educators, business and legal experts function as whole-person missionary teams, ministering to the needy at home and abroad. After completing their training, medical students and residents are expected to commit time to healing-team efforts. Compensation will be given in the form of tuition remission, as is presently done in certain Public Health Service programs and by many countries overseas.

Central to this educational process are the quality and spiritual commitment of the students and their faculty role models. At present, the schools of medicine, dentistry and nursing employ approximately one hundred basic science and clinical faculty, all of whom are dedicated Christians.

Symposium Outline
This collection of major presentations by ethicists, theologians and health-care professionals at the International Symposium on Whole-Person Medicine is divided into four sections.

The essays in Part I, "Toward a Whole-Person Perspective," present the philosophical basis for thinking in a wholistic paradigm: the Judeo-Christian faith requires commitment to a unified view of personhood connecting body, spirit, mind and environment.

Part II, "Medical Education," emphasizes that (1) a rigorous scientific approach must be an integral part of wholistic medicine for the continued development of innovative technologies and approaches for the care of persons; (2) the physician must have an awareness of his or her personal need for wholeness if the patient is to be treated wholistically; and (3) the time has come to discuss a conceptual framework for training the Christian physician.

The papers in Part III, "Models of Whole-Person Medicine," describe a variety of models endeavoring to use an integrative approach. Included are biblical models of medical care, church health-care clinics, care for the terminally ill and aspects of marriage and family life.

Part IV concludes the book with a chapter on "The Ministry of Medicine in the Care of the Whole Person" and the symposium's opening address, "A Clinical View of the Gospel."

Obviously this work is incomplete; the dimensions of the subject are almost infinite. We hope, however, that this collection will serve as a basis to stimulate thought, discussion and action. We are grateful to all those who made the symposium possible, including the faculty of the Oral Roberts University Medical School and the staff of the Christian Medical Society. Deserving special mention is Marsha Fowler, a Joseph P. Kennedy, Jr., Foundation Fellow in Medical Ethics at Harvard, who spent many hours editing and reorganizing the material.

David F. Allen
Lewis Penhall Bird
Robert Herrmann

Notes

[1]*New England Journal of Medicine* (8 February 1979).

[2]For simplicity all persons seeking health will be referred to as *patients,* recognizing that some such persons would normally be called *clients, counselees* or *consultees.*

[3]*Medicine* will be used in its broader sense to refer to health care that includes care by various professionals, not by physicians alone.

[4]J. H. Becker, *Het Begrip Nefesj in het O.T.* (1942); cited in G. C. Berkouwer, *Man: the Image of God,* trans. Dirk W. Jellema (Grand Rapids, Mich.: Eerdmans, 1962), p. 201.

[5]Berkouwer, p. 203.

[6]For a theological view of this issue see Berkouwer, above; for a psychological view see David G. Myers, *The Human Puzzle* (New York: Harper & Row, 1978), chap. 4, "Platonic Dualism or Hebraic Holism?"

[7]J. Barton Payne, *The Theology of the Older Testament* (Grand Rapids, Mich.: Zondervan Publishing House, 1962), p. 435.

Part I

Toward a Whole-Person Perspective in Medicine

Chapter One

Whole-Person Care: The Ethical Responsibility of the Physician

David F. Allen

Medicine has experienced two major revolutions and is now confronting a third.[1] The first was a movement from the religious-magical period to the ecological paradigm of Hippocratic medicine. The second was replacement of the Hippocratic ecological tradition by an emphasis on biomedical technology, still flourishing in our contemporary culture. Galdston argues that the third revolution will inaugurate a wholistic-ecological period.[2] After discussing these periods briefly I will examine the ethical responsibility of the health-care professional in the light of the present trend toward whole-person medicine.

Early Medicine: The Religious-Magical Period

The code of Hammurabi, the great Babylonian lawgiver (about 1950 B.C.), gives evidence of an organized medical profession among the Sumerians in the days of Abraham and indicates that medical and surgical practice was familiar to the Mesopotamians. The Babylonians knew how to prevent certain infectious diseases. The Assyrians had a pharmacopeia, and the Egyptians, through the practice of mummification, developed a detailed knowledge of human anatomy. The Egyptians and Assyrians laid a foundation on which the Greeks built.

Yet in spite of such practical skills, early medicine was a mixture of religious practice and magic. According to Garrison's treatise on the history of medicine, "the common point of convergence of all medical folklore is animism, . . . the notion that the world swarms with invisible spirits which are the efficient causes of disease and death."[3]

In animism, the workings of nature were assumed to be visible manifestations of malevolent gods, demons, spirits and other supernatural agents. Thus disease was (1) the work of an evil spirit or other deities who were to be cajoled or placated by burnt offerings and sacrifices, or (2) the product of a human enemy with supernatural powers, or (3) the action of an offended spirit of dead human beings, animals or plants.[4]

Consequently, the doctor/healer/witch doctor/medicine man/shaman assumed a supervisory relationship to the disease and its cure. Medical treatment meant (1) using quasi-psychotherapeutic methods to induce autosuggestion in the client, (2) frightening demons away by shouts, costumes, etc., and (3) capitalizing on the suggestive power of fetishes or amulets worn by the patient. Treatment was often thought to be more effective if accompanied by song and dance.

The purely magical perspective was rejected by certain religious groups, especially the Hebrews. The Hebrews knew God as a dependable God, not as a capricious Being whose will could be assuaged through spell or sacrifice. For example, the Hebrew prophet Micah, speaking from the countryside of the southern kingdom set between the great empires of Egypt and Assyria, could say, "What doth the LORD require of thee, but to do justly, and to love mercy, and to walk humbly with thy God?" (Mic. 6:8 KJV).

According to Garlick, "In spite of the limitations of early Jewish thought, its spiritual approach to health was nevertheless a vital contribution to the medical art."[5]

Mosaic Law, a religious-ethical legal system, contained many elements that safeguarded Hebrew health. By their code of ritual hygiene, the Jewish priests effectively became public health officers. Moreover, the religious observance of one day's rest in seven had an important bearing on the health of the community. It has been argued that the Hebrew approach to health opened the way for the next major medical movement.

Hippocratic Ecological Period

The more organized scientific approach of the Greeks was personified by Hippocrates.[6] Born in 460 B.C., he trained in Greek medical schools which drew upon Egyptian, Persian and Indian sources. Without knowledge of anatomy and physiology to guide him, Hippocrates learned to depend on observation and the healing power of nature, thus liberating investigation and treatment of disease from magic and superstition.

His dictum, "To know is science but merely to believe one knows is ignorance," became the basis of scientific medicine. His observation of and respect for the vital balance in nature led to many valid medical discoveries, including malarial fever, epilepsy, dysentery, melancholia and mania. He instituted careful, systematic examination of the patient's facial appearance, pulse, temperature, respiration and body movements. He categorized disease as acute or chronic and introduced the doctrine of the four "humors" and healing by primary intention. The Hippocratic oath, derived from the Hippocratic corpus, laid the basis for medical ethics up to the present day.

For Hippocrates, accord with nature resulted in health; discord resulted in disease. Thus he insisted, "Nature heals; the physician is only nature's assistant." That ecological perspective underscored the importance of a harmonious interdependence of human beings and nature. Rather than isolate disease for examination as a special problem, it focused on the patient in his or her natural environment. Thus patients were seen as major contributors to their disease, depending on their lifestyle. The Hippocratic Tract of Ancient Medicine (about 430-420 B.C.) states, "There would have been no need for medicine if sick men had profited from the same mode of living and regimen of food and drink as men in health."[7]

Until the sixteenth century the Hippocratic tradition had supreme authority in all European and Islamic countries. Though the Judeo-Christian concept of God replaced the Ionian view of *physis* (nature) as the core of the universe, the Hippocratic perspective of ecological interdependence remained intact.[8]

Supernatural healing by God was not ignored, however. Believing Christ to be present through the Holy Spirit, the church effected his ministry through various spiritual gifts, including the gift of healing. Such gifts were backed up by a praying, caring body of believers. The corporate faith and concern of the Christian community inspired the early church as a healing body.

On the natural level, biblical practices often paralleled the ecological Hippocratic tradition. For example, the use of wine and oil was common in Greek medicine (1 Tim. 5:23; Jas. 5:14). Patristic writings (Justin Martyr, Irenaeus, Tertullian, Clement of Alexandria and Origen) also contain references to Greek medical techniques.

The emphasis on healing in the Christian community made caring for the sick a sacred obligation. Pastoral and medical care was undertaken by bishops and presbyters; deacons and deaconesses visited the sick in their homes. That stood in contrast with the attitude toward sickness and misfortune prevalent at that time, which was "not one of compassion ... the credit of ministering to human suffering on an extended scale belongs to Christians."[9]

Once Christianity became the state religion, care of the sick was instituted on a larger scale. Tradition credits Helena, Constantine's mother, with beginning the movement to establish Christian hospitals.[10] In A.D. 369, Basil of Caesarea formed the first hospital for lepers. In 375 Ephraem and his Nestorian followers offered three hundred beds for plague victims at Edessa in Mesopotamia. Twenty-four years later Chupostam began a "hospital" for the poor in Byzantium. In the fifth century the first general hospital in the West was established in Rome by a woman named Fabiola. According to Jerome, its purpose was "to gather in the sick from the streets and to nurse wretched sufferers, wasted with poverty and disease."[11]

After the fall of the Roman Empire, the church-organized network of health care collapsed. During the middle ages monasteries became the centers of health care and medical learning. In character, however, medicine was still in the Hippocratic tradition. For example, in the sixth century Cassiodorus established a monastery in southern Italy and stated in the rule:

> I insist, brothers, that those who treat the health of the brethren . . . should fulfill their duties with exemplary piety. . . . Let them serve with sincere study to help those that are ailing, as becomes their knowledge of medicine, and let them look for their reward from Him who compensates temporal work by eternal wages. Learn, therefore, the nature of herbs, and study diligently the way to combine their various species for human health, but do not place your entire hope on herbs, nor seek to restore health only by human counsels. Since medicine has been created by God and since it is He who gives back health and restores life, turn to Him.[12]

Tragically, later authorities of the church sought to suppress experimental science. In the sixth century Emperor Justinian I closed the medical schools of Athens and Alexandria. In 1123 the Lateran Council under Pope Calixtus II forbade both the religious and secular clergy to attend to the sick, other than to serve as spiritual directors. The same edict was confirmed by Innocent II at the Council of Rheims in 1131. In 1215 Innocent III condemned surgery and in 1248 dissection was declared to be sacrilegious. Underlying those developments was a theological belief that the body was the prison of the soul and was of little importance for the spiritual well-being of the person. Nevertheless medicine continued to flourish in spite of great difficulty. Introduction of "physic gardens" in the monasteries led to a closer union between medicine and nature, re-emphasizing the Hippocratic tradition. Oddly enough, the Nestorians, followers of Nestorius (who was declared a heretic by the church) continued to spread Greek medicine to the wider world. Their school at

Edessa played a significant part in the Arabic revival of learning which deeply influenced the cultural life of Europe and opened the way for the Renaissance.

Biomedical Period

At the time of the Renaissance a growing separation of medicine and religion was accentuated as freedom of inquiry flourished in secular society. Copernicus in 1543 propounded his theory of a heliocentric universe, which was followed a year later by the evidence from Galileo's telescope. The revelation that the known physical world was but a particle of an infinite universe revolutionized the ancient concept of the world and enlarged the bounds of science. The science of Copernicus and Galileo challenged the theories of Aristotle and Ptolemy. When the experimental method was applied to dissecting the human body, the views of Hippocrates, Aristotle and Galen were contradicted.

In the year of the Copernican revolution, 1543, Vesalius published *Fabrica,* a thorough analysis of the human body based on meticulous dissection. As the founder of modern anatomy, Vesalius restored to the world of medicine the ancient Greek principle of organized and systematic observation. An intense desire to know, beyond mere reliance on nature, started to ring the death knell of the Hippocratic tradition.

In the seventeenth century, the "Golden Age of mathematicians, astronomers and physicists," the experimental method was effectively established in medicine through the brilliant work of the English physician William Harvey by his discovery of the circulation of the blood. Hence Vesalius disclosed the structure of the human body, and Harvey, following his tradition, led the way to the study of its functioning. By laying the basis of experimental science, the two men led the medical renaissance and brought to an end 1,400 years of written authority.[13]

It is difficult to pinpoint exactly what caused the biomedical revolution[14] or to determine why the Hippocratic ecological paradigm disappeared. We do know, however, that with industrialization and the ensuing growth of the habitable world came the onset of crowd diseases. Those diseases, caused by bacterial and viral agents, were endemic and epidemic, affecting whole populations. The Hippocratic tradition, which depended on a stable ecology, rural economy and often an individual approach, was ineffective against the new diseases, and in time Hippocratic medicine was abandoned.

In its place the biomedical experimental model, stressing the need to understand causation, led to significant medical discoveries: Jenner's cowpox vaccine (1798), Pasteur's discovery of bacteria and Lister's antiseptic principle. Application of Pasteur's bacteriological discoveries to tropical medicine led to the etiology of leprosy, tetanus, plague, typhoid, tuberculosis, cholera, malaria and yellow fever. Beyond conquering the epidemic diseases such as smallpox and tuberculosis, inroads were made into the deficiency diseases (pellagra, beriberi, kwashiorkor) and such psychiatrically associated syndromes as hysteria. Along with ability to diagnose the basic cause of diseases with microbial-viral etiologies has come development of a therapeutic armamentarium of powerful drugs including antibiotics, psychotropic medication, insulin for diabetes and vitamin B-12 for pernicious anemia.

It is of particular note that during that period much emphasis was placed on medical missions. Yale's Peter Parker trained in medicine and religion, organized medical missions in China and was instrumental in creating international awareness of the health needs of less privileged peoples. That led to the establishment of medical missions in Africa, Asia and South America. Moreover, John Wesley and other renowned evangelists practiced medicine during their missions. Wesley established the first free medical dispensary in England in 1746, aiming his work at the poor (who were neglected by the medical profession because they could not afford to pay).

In a letter to the Rev. Vincent Perronet, Wesley wrote: "But I was still in pain for many of the poor that were sick: there was so great expense and so little profit.... I then asked the advice of several physicians for them, but still it profitted not. I saw the poor people paining away and several families ruined and that without remedy."[15]

The wholistic tradition was common in the United States where Congregational ministers like Cotton Mather saw physical healing as a part of their ministry. Mather's work on inoculation resulted in many scholars acclaiming him "the first significant figure in American medicine."[16] Then as late as 1860 a Congregational minister in Guilford, Connecticut, collaborated with a physician in preparing a family medical journal.

In spite of its rich religious heritage, European and American medicine evolved separately from the church. The reasons for that are inconclusive. But the breakup of the medical system at the time of the Reformation and Renaissance, the influence of the mind-body dualism of Descartes in the seventeenth century and the later influence of positivism are all contributory.

Toward a Wholistic Ecological Revolution

A purely biomedical model assumes that disease is due primarily to anatomic and physiological aberrations. Thus the task of the physician is to diagnose the abnormalities associated with disease and use technology to restore them to a normal state. According to Engel, "In modern Western society biomedicine not only has provided a basis for the scientific study of disease, it has also become our own culturally specific perspective about disease, that is, our folk model. Indeed, the biomedical model is now the dominant folk model of disease in the Western world."[17]

With increased knowledge about disease, medicine has grown in complexity and dependence on expensive diagnostic and therapeutic technology. That, in turn, has forced specialization and reduced the emphasis on wholistic care. Some medical theorists argue that the human dimension is being lost from medical care. Ironically, in becoming experts at treating disease we may have forgotten how to treat persons.

In spite of the success of biomedical technology, a new revolution is upon us. That is because a purely biomedical model is limited in confronting many serious challenges to contemporary health care. A few examples of such challenges include the following.

1. *Personal responsibility for health.* Increasing evidence shows that the health of human beings is determined primarily by their behavior, nutrition and the nature of their environment. According to Dr. John Knowles, late president of the Rockefeller Foundation:

> Prevention of disease means forsaking the bad habits which many people enjoy—overeating, too much drinking, taking pills, staying up at night, engaging in promiscuous sex, driving too fast and smoking cigarettes—or, put another way, it means doing things which require special effort—exercising regularly, going to the dentist, practicing contraception, ensuring harmonious family life, submitting to screening examinations.[18]

Studies by Breslow and Belloc of nearly 7,000 adults followed for 5½ years showed that life expectancy and health are significantly related to the following basic health habits:

> three meals a day at regular times and no snacking
> breakfast every day
> moderate exercise two or three times a week
> adequate sleep (seven or eight hours a night)
> no smoking
> moderate weight
> no alcohol or only in moderation[19]

A forty-five-year-old man who practices up to three of these habits has a remaining life expectancy of 21.6 years (to age 67 years). A man with six or seven of these habits has a life expectancy of 33.1 years (to age 78). Thus eleven years could be added to life expectancy by simple changes in habits of living. This is especially impressive since life expectancy at age 65 increased by only 2.7 years during the period between 1900 and 1966.

Evidence is beginning to show that a large percentage of deaths due to cardiovascular disease and cancer are occurring in young individuals and are related to lifestyle habits. Heart disease and strokes are related to diet, smoking, undetected hypertension and lack of exercise. Cancer, on the other hand, is related to smoking and perhaps to a diet rich in fats and refined foodstuffs and low in residue. Cancer may also result from ingestion of food additives and certain drugs or the inhalation of a wide variety of noxious agents. A smaller fraction may be due to occupational exposures and personal hygienic factors.

It is not my intention to introduce a new health puritanism or to go back to the days of judgmental attitudes resulting in such diagnoses as "moral turpitude." I wish, rather, to stress the need for a wholistic ecological approach that focuses on health and its maintenance rather than solely on disease and its treatment.

2. *Problems of specific populations.* We are particularly challenged by the specific needs of such populations as children, adolescents and the elderly.

The breakdown of the family, along with the inefficiency and inadequate nurturing ability of many day-care centers, places many children at risk. Living in an environment with little stability, consistency and predictability, they are in need of a wholistic support system. Fraiberg postulates that without such, their capacity to develop intimacy is diminished and they withdraw into themselves, becoming what she terms "hollow people" who are indifferent to life and unable to relate to other humans.[20] Of particular note is the need for supportive services to single parents who must work, run the home and provide the nurture of both father and mother. In many urban and suburban areas, lack of support makes such an experience a nightmare for parent and child.

Child abuse is a major problem. Its cause evades us. But the challenge of its prevention demands the full attention of health-care resources. Obviously good biomedical technology alone is not enough.

Teen-age pregnancy now haunts us. In the past ten years, while births to women over nineteen years have decreased, births to girls under nineteen have increased by fifty per cent.

Because of poor prenatal care and nutrition a high percentage of those children are born prematurely with a tendency to develop learning disabilities, mental retardation and other disorders. Moreover, if the young girls do not return to school or other vocational development, eighty per cent of them will have a repeat pregnancy within five years. Yet the Johns Hopkins center for teen-age pregnancy has demonstrated that wholistic care including health education, long-term follow-up and vocational counseling leads to more responsible attitudes toward relationships, reduced prematurity rate and higher-quality parenting.[21]

Another major public-health problem is the issue of adolescent violence, which accounts for the majority of deaths of black teen-agers, inhumane harassment of the elderly and lack of safety in our parks and neighborhoods. It is a societal responsibility (as yet unaddressed), which requires a multi-disciplinary approach including input from the health-care perspective.

Though persons are living longer physiologically, because of the lack and inaccessibility of support systems, we may be dying earlier sociologically. Therefore we need a health-care model beyond the purely biomedical mode to bring hope and caring to the elderly, who are making up an ever-increasing proportion of our population.

3. *Need for mediating structures in health care.* The sudden but gigantic growth of the health/human-services bureaucracy demands the specialization of health professionals and a new sophistication on the part of the consumer. The fact is that many of our consumers, including children, adolescents, the elderly and persons who are mentally retarded or chronically mentally ill, find it difficult to negotiate their own services. With the breakdown of the extended and nuclear family and the transitory nature of neighborhoods and communities, many persons have no advocate. They languish without care, even though services are available. Peter Berger, a leading sociologist, says that the health-care megastructure desperately needs mediating structures to act between it and the consumer. Such structures would enhance utilization,

provide advocacy, curtail abuses and encourage reform.[22] He argues that the religious community (church and synagogue), one of the remaining transgenerational communities in the culture, could provide powerful advocacy and support services for many at-risk clients (the elderly, children, chronic patients and others).

To meet such challenges, more than a purely biomedical model is needed. Thus a third revolution, the change to an ecological-wholistic approach to health care, is appearing on the horizon. It is not a return to the Hippocratic-ecological tradition, a simplistic reductionism impossible in our time. Rather, the ethical, social, legal and psychological challenges facing health care are moving beyond the purely biomedical perspective to develop a wholistic model that will encompass the total functioning of persons and their relationships with each other and with their environment.

The Ethical Responsibility of the Health-Care Professional[23]

In light of the wholistic ecological challenges facing us, what is the ethical responsibility of the health-care professional? Referring to Ralph Potter's paradigm for an ethical analysis of social policy, the following categories should be examined: the facts, theological or quasi-theological assumptions, moral reasoning, and implementation.[24]

Facts

Good ethics demand good data. Therefore it is important that we seriously commit ourselves to master the body of knowledge of our particular discipline. Good preparatory training, meaningful continuing education, and relevant, well-organized research are essential for ethical decision making.

Firth's Ideal Observer Theory is a particularly useful model to help us conceptualize our commitment to fact finding. According to Firth, the Ideal Observer should be omniscient, omnipercipient, disinterested and dispassionate, consistent and otherwise normal.[25] Although those characteristics are impossible to achieve in an absolute sense, they enable us to focus our ambitions.

Being omniscient. Beyond the commitment to master the body of knowledge of our particular field, wholistic medicine requires that we learn about other disciplines that influence the care of our clients. Wholistic medicine implies having an integrated perspective of the personal, social, psychological, spiritual, ethical, cultural and political influences on the patient's life. Obviously one cannot be an expert in all fields, but it is important that we learn to consult experts in other fields and work with them in healing teams.

Being omnipercipient. A wholistic approach requires that we extend ourselves to understand how the client perceives his or her pain. To approach omnipercipience, the physician should try to understand how his or her work is perceived by and affects others. This requires a humane sensitivity to the patient's perspective and feelings about the illness, treatment process or research.

The dynamic principle here is "empathic caring"—which results from identifying with others and then treating them as you would want to be treated. In essence, it is the principle of reciprocity better known as the Golden Rule.

Putting the principle of reciprocity into practice, however, demands a marked degree of psychological maturity, including an ability to imagine the hurt of others vividly and a willingness to be open and tolerant. I don't want to imply that all physicians should have psychotherapy to improve their personalities; I do believe, however, that doctors should be honest in asking themselves if they can relate to their patients. If they cannot, then I suggest some form of therapy or learning experience to enhance their ability to empathize with the people they serve. For example, a group of colleagues at Boston City Hospital, realizing their inability to communicate effectively with the many community groups served by the hospital, organized mutual educational seminars for doctors and consumers. It was a challenging learning experience for both groups and had a positive effect on the overall delivery of health care.

Although learning experiences may result in increased self-knowledge or community awareness on the part of the doctor, often the needed step is of the most rudimentary nature: for example, learning how to speak Spanish when one has Hispanic patients.

Being disinterested and dispassionate. The Ideal Observer is disinterestedly interested and dispassionately passionate. I suggest that a relative state of disinterestedness and dispassionateness can be achieved through a multidisciplinary review committee in the decision-making process. Thus particular interests or passions are diluted and balanced by those who hold opposing views or perspectives. Multidisciplinary committees can offer broader-based advocacy and insure informed consent. Such a committee is supportive of both the physician and the patient and simultaneously provides a mutual educational experience and communications channel. This engenders an atmosphere of trust and openness within the doctor-patient relationship, which leads to the delivery of more just and humane medical care.

Being consistent. Being consistent does not mean a rigid, inflexible attitude, but rather implies sincere commitment to the fair treatment of all individuals regardless of their cultural or socioeconomic background. This is particularly relevant in a wholistic approach, which recognizes a multidimensional view of the person. For example, although medical treatment is often unable to provide a cure for mental retardation, taking certain social-technological approaches toward the person and his or her environment may produce a better life for that person.

Being otherwise normal—recognizing limitations. Finally, the Ideal Observer should be otherwise "normal." Even after making every effort in the patient's best interests, the doctor is a person with limited knowledge and expertise. Any expert is periodically subject to failure through ignorance, oversight or incompetence, especially when complex medical problems and informed consent are involved. Awareness of limitation and possible failure should not cause doctors to retreat, but should underscore their responsibility to recognize their limitations and allow their work to be examined in an atmosphere of openness and consultation with others, both inside and outside their discipline.

Theological Basis

Good medical practice requires more than accurate information and technical competence. Facts and technical knowledge must be related to the human ethical perspective in order to serve the best interests of the patient. According to Arieti, "Values always accompany and give special psychological significance to facts . . . when we deprive facts of their value, we fabricate artifacts which have no reality in human psychology. An individual may suspend his value judgment when he wants to examine a fact from a specific point of view, but then the ethical content has to be re-established if the fact is to have human significance. If we remove the ethical dimension, we reduce man to subhuman animal."[26]

Physicians must be cognizant of their personal ethical value system and its relation to those they serve. One's belief about the nature of human beings exerts a subtle but controlling influence on attitudes, behavior and treatment of individuals. Eisenberg says, "What we believe of men affects the behavior of man, for it determines what each expects from each other. Theories of education, of political science and economics and the very policies of government are based on implied concepts of the nature of man."[27]

Returning to the principle of reciprocity mentioned earlier, it is quite evident that physicians cannot apply the Golden Rule in their work if they do not believe that other people deserve the same dignity, respect and medical treatment they want for themselves and their families. For example, during an evaluation of a community mental-health center, a psychiatrist commented that "even though the state hospital environment is substandard, it's suitable for chronic mentally ill patients because they don't need anything better." Obviously, such a value system affects that man's attitude and treatment of chronically ill patients and hence his commitment to mental-health reform.

For the most part, Western ethics are based on the Judeo-Christian tradition which, at its heart, claims that human beings are made in the image of God (Gen. 1:27). Although human beings are alienated from their Creator, and experience the painful ambiguity of good and evil in their existence, the atoning death and victorious resurrection of Christ witness to the triumphant meaning of the individual. Christ came to redeem the tarnished *imago dei* which, however marred, is the basis for personhood, dignity and basic human rights. A sense of the inestimable value of the individual enhances personal meaning, interpersonal relationships and human community. It is that reverence for human life that Niebuhr says is necessary for meaningful social reform.[28]

All individuals, regardless of sex, age, race, class or illness are persons first, deserving the utmost respect and concern. The basis for the doctor-patient relationship, therefore, is mutual God-given personhood and human dignity. Buber draws a distinction between the I-Thou relationship and the dehumanized I-it or subject-object interaction. The reciprocal ability to see in each other the person, the shared human qualities which go deeper than any differences, is the essential ingredient for truly informed consent and a trusting relationship between patient and health professional.

In addition to the empathy and accurate information transmitted through the doctor-patient relationship, a sound theological-ethical base includes forgiveness, truth telling, love, promise keeping, justice, liberty and noninjury. Those principles are so germane to the entire human community that they may be called the constitutive imperatives—that is, the underlying principles on which all laws governing human society (not just the doctor-patient relationship) are made.

Jonsen and Butler emphasize the importance of this concept: "Respect for individuals requires that every individual be treated in consideration of his uniqueness, equal to every other, and that special justification is required for interference with their purposes, their privacy or their behavior. It implies sets of liberties, rights and duties and obligations, especially of promise-keeping and truth-telling."[29]

In a whole-person medicine paradigm, a sense of community requires that we place ourselves in the position of the client and treat him or her as we would wish to be treated. The ethical dynamic is that if the treatment or research process would not be acceptable for the physician or his family, neither would it be suitable for the client.

Moral Reasoning

The moral reasoning underlying any decision-making process affects the way persons are treated. Physicians must therefore examine the types of moral reasoning operating in their work and the way they approach the question of informed consent. Forms of moral reasoning range from ethical egoism (as in Kohlberg's moral development Stage I) to a more sophisticated formalism (as in Kohlberg's Stage VI).[30] In my experience, the physician is most often confronted by two major conflicting types of moral reasoning: the social-utility *versus* the equal-value view of life.

Though the concept of social utility comes in many varieties, its essence can be summed up as promoting the greatest good for the greatest number or for the most powerful (who define what constitutes utility). Though appealing to the majority or to the most powerful, this philosophy offers little for those who are in the minority or without power. When unchecked, this "for the good of humanity" motivation has led to atrocities inflicted by biomedical technology on certain disadvantaged groups—the mentally ill, the mentally retarded, the elderly, the racially outcast—groups assumed expendable in calculating greater good. Naturally, informed consent from those in the minority group is considered relatively unimportant and is either ignored entirely or obtained deceitfully.

Underlying the social-utility concept is the assumption that only life of a certain "quality" or usefulness has worth. Thus there is a tendency to define personhood on the basis of an individual's relative social utility. Whenever the person's utility/disutility ratio is low, that individual's worth as a person is assumed to be low. Being mentally retarded, for example, reduces utility. As a result, the person becomes subject to a bar-rage of indignities and loss of human rights, manifested by dehumanizing living conditions, unethical research, poor medical treatment and inadequate education.

Once persons are rated according to their social utility, the merit view of justice will deny certain persons positive pre-sumption, due process and equality—all under the euphe-mism of maximizing the public good. This strains the moral fiber of the society itself. Utility must never define person-hood and the right to life, liberty and good in the world. Jus-tice demands equal consideration of each person's claim, re-gardless of the person and his or her situation or power base in society.

The powerful in society must share their power with those who have none, making advantages for even those who are most disadvantaged. We would do well to remember that the disadvantaged are an integral part of human society. They are a part of us and we are a part of them. The way we treat them is a direct reflection of the quality of existence we es-pouse. Therefore, physicians must be guardians of the hu-man ethical dynamic in society. That can be done effectively only if the moral reasoning implicit in their work leads to the enhancement of the dignity of all persons, especially those in need.

Loyalties dictate the ultimate ends we serve and the means we employ in our work. "For where your treasure is, there will your heart be also" (Mt. 6:21). One of the most important ends for the physician in addition to providing sound medical care is to allow patients to experience the meaning and fulfill-ment of their God-given personhood, dignity and human rights. All else, even the informed-consent process, is pri-marily a means to that end. In order to help individuals appre-ciate their own worth and dignity, however, the doctor must also be committed to the broader responsibility of fighting for more equitable justice structures in the surrounding society.

A clear perspective of means and ends is of utmost impor-tance. Whenever means become ends in themselves, persons are affected—they are dehumanized or even destroyed. In medicine this is especially true, as we saw demonstrated in the Holocaust. The medical practices of German physicians led to the degradation and destruction of human life and values rather than to any respect for them.[31] This means-as-ends perspective produced a "radical evil" that will never be rectified but must be prevented from recurring.

A more contemporary example is the recent trend of deinstitutionalization of chronically mentally ill patients. At times deinstitutionalization, an excellent means to achieve the end of good patient care for some persons, becomes an end in itself. Rather than increasing human dignity and well-being, irresponsible deinstitutionalization leaves some persons to fend for themselves in deplorable living conditions with no proper follow-up care. Likewise, it is possible to obtain good informed consent and yet deliver shoddy medical care or perform sloppy, unethical research. The physician should also be aware that at times informed consent may be difficult to obtain; yet, this must not affect his or her commitment to act in the patient's best interests. Faced with that commitment, one may have to refuse to conduct research on certain "consenting" populations (for example, prisoners or children), decide on the need for further consultation, or even choose emergency intervention to save a person's life when informed consent has been impossible to obtain. The physician's primary commitment is to the welfare of patients as full members of the human community.

Implementation of Wholistic Health Care
To counteract the possibility of wholistic medicine becoming empty rhetoric, or just another fad, we must emphasize particular proposals for action.

1. *Clarification of our convictions and motivation for whole-person medicine.* This can be done by asking ourselves such questions as: Am I treating my patients as I would want myself or family to be treated? How can my interaction with my patients enhance their personal meaning and individuality? Have I explored multidimensional aspects of my patients' lives? Have I

sought to understand their problems? How do they feel about my intervention?

2. *"Cross-fertilized" education.* In order to develop effective and competent healing teams, "cross-fertilized" graduate education in human services is urgently needed. Such programs must be well organized and thoroughly evaluated. The overall goal should be to enable multidisciplinary professionals including lawyers, doctors, social workers, businesspeople and so on, to talk with each other about human needs. Particular issues to comprise the curriculum include: models of human development and functioning, including emotional, cultural, social, economic aspects; group-process issues; health education and nutrition, physical fitness and so on.

3. *Comprehensive health education.* Whole-person medicine requires exposure to health education in all areas of society including school, neighborhood and church. This requires full support of the government and the voluntary agencies of society.

4. *Organization of mediating structures.* According to Berger, in view of the burgeoning megasphere of human services, there is an urgent need for effective mediating structures.[32] Acting on behalf of the individual, such structures should provide advocacy, information about services, health education and supportive community to enhance the effectiveness and humanization of the human-service bureaucracy.

5. *Better coordination and linkage of local human-service programs.* The splintering, defensiveness and lack of coordination of local community-health programs impedes wholistic delivery of health care. This is particularly noticeable in services for adolescent and elderly populations who require comprehensive programs. The effectiveness of such programs as the DOOR program for adolescents in New York is noteworthy.

6. *Need for community.* In light of the breakdown of the family and the transient nature of our neighborhood populations there is an urgent need for supportive communities for children, families, adolescents, handicapped persons and the elderly. Familiar though we are with the concept of com-

munity health and community mental health, in reality there is little community. Community requires a base for communion, a base that enhances communication and mutual sharing. The church, with the powerful meaning of the Eucharist, offers such a base and hence a revitalization of community. The establishment of wholistic-health clinics in churches and the appointment of human-services professionals to work in churches are promising signs.

Notes

[1] I. Galdston, "The Third Revolution: Prelude and Polemic," in *Ethical Issues in Medicine: The Role of the Physician in Today's Society,* ed. E. Fuller Torrey (Boston: Little, Brown & Co., 1968), p. 18.

[2] Ibid.; J. Jekel, "The Coming Revolution in Health Care," paper presented at a national meeting of the American Scientific Affiliation (Nyack, N.Y.: 14 August 1977).

[3] F. H. Garrison, *History of Medicine,* 4th ed. (Philadelphia: W. B. Saunders, 1929), pp. 20-21.

[4] Ibid.

[5] P. L. Garlick, *Man's Search for Health: A Study in the Interrelation of Religion and Medicine* (London: Highway Press, 1952), p. 29.

[6] Galdston, p. 5.

[7] W. H. S. Jones, ed., *Hippocrates,* I (Cambridge, Mass.: Harvard Univ. Press, 1923), pp. 13-63.

[8] Galdston, p. 7.

[9] Garrison, p. 178.

[10] I am indebted to Scott Morris, a graduate of Yale Divinity School and presently a student at Yale University School of Medicine, for an understanding of this historical perspective.

[11] Garlick, p. 191.

[12] Ibid., p. 211.

[13] Ibid., p. 50.

[14] H. Rasmussen, *Pharos,* 38 (1975), 53.

[15] A. Wesley Hill, *John Wesley Among the Physicians* (London: Epworth Press, 1958).

[16] Otto Beall, *Cotton Mather: First Significant Figure in American Medicine* (Baltimore: Johns Hopkins, 1954), p. 126.

[17] G. Engel, "The Need for a New Medical Model: A Challenge for Biomedicine," *Science,* 196, No. 4286 (8 April 1977).

[18] J. Knowles, "The Responsibility of the Individual," *Daedalus* (Winter 1977), p. 65.

[19] N. B. Belloc and L. Breslow, "The Relation of Physical Health States and Health Practices," *Preventive Medicine,* I (August 1972), 409-21. See also "The Relationship of Health Practices and Mortality," *Preventive Medicine,*

2 (1973), 67-81.

[20]Selma Fraiberg, *Every Child's Birthright: In Defense of Mothering* (New York: Bantam, 1979).

[21]David F. Allen, Family Development Plan submitted to H.E.W. Secretary Joseph Califano, April 1977.

[22]P. Berger, *To Empower People: Role of Mediating Structures in Public Policy* (Washington, D.C.: American Enterprise Institute for Public Policy Research, 1977). For a discussion of other serious challenges to the reigning biomedical paradigm see Professor James Jekel's chapter in this compendium (pp. 121-51). He examines such challenges as an over-estimation of the biomedical impact, the prevailing emphasis on disease as opposed to health, iatrogenesis (side effects of medication, abuse of Valium, etc.) and increasing costs of health care.

[23]Certain aspects of this discussion appeared in an article, "The Ethical Responsibility of the Physician," *Yale Journal of Biology and Medicine,* 9, No. 5 (November 1976).

[24]Ralph Potter, *War and Moral Discourse* (Richmond, Va.: John Knox Press, 1969), pp. 23-24.

[25]Roderick Firth, "Ethical Absolutism and the Ideal Observer," *Philosophy and Phenomenological Research,* 12, No. 3 (1952), 317-45.

[26]S. Arieti, "Psychiatric Controversy: Man's Ethical Dimension," *American Journal of Psychiatry,* 132 (1975), 1.

[27]Leon Eisenberg, "The Human Nature of Human Nature," *Science,* 176 (1972), pp. 124.

[28]Reinhold Niebuhr, *Moral Man and Immoral Society* (New York: Scribner's, 1932), pp. 58-59.

[29]A. Jonsen and L. Butler, "Public Ethics and Policy Making," *Hastings Center Report,* 5, No. 4 (1965), 25.

[30]L. Kohlberg, "The Claim to Moral Adequacy of a Highest Stage of Moral Judgment," *Journal of Philosophy,* 70 (1973), 630-46.

[31]L. Alexander, "Science Under Dictatorship," *New England Journal of Medicine,* 241 (1949), 39-47.

[32]Berger, pp. 1-7.

Chapter Two

An Ethic of the
Healing Art

Arthur J. Dyck

The art of healing is an art of helping persons. Healing is not merely something that happens to bodies. It is an event in the life of a person as a whole. This conference on whole-person medicine is rightly asking us to consider how we should practice medicine that aims to heal the whole person.

Our society and the medical professions are presently exhibiting considerable concern about the nature and definition of personhood. Not all of that concern is in my judgment advantageous to patients.

One glaring example of what I have in mind is found in the criterion and practice reported by Duff and Campbell of Yale University.[1] With the consent of the families in question, Duff and Campbell make decisions that certain infants should not receive the life-saving medical intervention they need. Why? Because, as they say, "such very defective individuals were considered to have little or no hope of achieving meaningful 'humanhood.' "[2] For support they cite an Episcopalian minister, an ethicist, Joseph Fletcher, and his article "Indicators of Humanhood."[3] In a more recent publication, a Roman Catholic theologian, Richard McCormick, insists that we need intervene to save the lives only of those who have potential for human relationships.[4] Duff and Campbell describe as below the threshhold of humanhood an infant "who has little or no capacity to love or be loved."[5] Notice the qualification *"little capacity."* One wonders how much and how measurable is "little." Certainly Duff and Campbell are willing to consign to their death Down's Syndrome infants, who are generally very loving and lovable children. Earlier, Joseph Fletcher had written, "A Down's is not a person."[6]

One of the most devastating responses to the Duffs and Campbells of this world came in a letter to the editor of *Newsweek.* The letter was written in response to a *Newsweek* article describing the work of Duff and Campbell.

> I'll wager my entire root systems and as much fertilizer as it would take to fill Yale University that you never received a letter from a vegetable before this one; but, much as I resent the term, I must confess that I fit the description of a "vegetable" as defined in the article "Shall this Child Die?"
>
> Due to severe brain damage incurred at birth, I am unable to dress myself, toilet myself, or write; my secretary is typing this letter. Many thousands of dollars had to be spent on my rehabilitation and education in order for me to reach my present professional status as a counseling psychologist. My parents were also told, 35 years ago, that there was little or no hope of achieving meaningful "humanhood" for their daughter. Have I reached "humanhood"? Compared with Drs. Duff and Campbell, I believe I have surpassed it!
>
> Instead of changing the law to make it legal to weed out us "vegetables," let us change the laws so that we may receive quality medical care, education and freedom to live as full and productive lives as our potentials will allow.[7]

I begin, therefore, with a sober warning that we not invent concepts or definitions of personhood that may be used to deprive human beings, members of the human species, of their usual rights to life, liberty and the pursuit of happiness; nor should we invent a notion of personhood that undermines the basic equality of every human being, regardless of age, sex, color, social and economic status or physical condition. Human beings deserve to be treated as persons in every aspect of their being. What I wish to examine, therefore, are the moral norms that ought to govern our care and concern for human beings as whole persons.

I will use three basic concepts to elucidate the parameters of medical care that would constitute care for the whole person. First, there is compassion, which affirms our respect for all human beings as persons having worth in themselves. Second, there is covenant, which affirms our respect for human beings as persons having worth in relation to us and to others. Third, there is community, which affirms human beings as persons worthy in relation to the whole moral universe in all of its power and reality.

Compassion

In dictionaries, compassion is defined as an attitude with two components: deep sympathy for the suffering or trouble of others, accompanied by an urge to help. Sympathy inclines us not only to help but to refrain from injuring others or from causing them any kind of suffering. Compassion is at the heart of the most fundamental motives and practical guides for giving medical care: to help, but first of all, to do no harm.

Human beings are living organisms. A fundamental, constitutive rule guiding our behavior toward such living organisms is the injunction not to kill. What is a constitutive rule? At the very least, it is a rule without which we consider rule making to be impractical or even impossible. Who would contemplate forming or entering into a society indifferent to the value of human life and unwilling to protect it? Here we see one of the rational underpinnings of the Ten Commandments found in Jewish and Christian Scriptures. In the same Scriptures, the Ten Commandments are said to be summarized by love for neighbor and for God. To refrain from killing is a form of love or compassion.

Concern for the whole person begins, therefore, with commitment to the value of technical skills in medicine. One of my students, a medical doctor at Mass. General Hospital, underlined that critical dimension of compassion in a recent paper.[8] She reported that one of her cardiac patients once remarked: "It's fine if the doctor is a nice guy, but what I'm here for is a new heart valve." She then went on to raise a significant ques-

tion: How much would we value more compassionate physicians if to be more compassionate would mean to be less skillful?

> Cardiac surgery mortalities for three Boston hospitals were
> recently listed in the *Boston Globe:* 5% mortality at the big,
> impersonal academic center, 10% at the pleasant, middle-
> sized community hospital staffed with surgeons from the
> big, impersonal academic center, 40% at the small-to-
> middle-sized, non-academic, community hospital. What is
> ambience worth in per cent mortality?[9]

Compassion for whole persons begins with conscientious mas-
tery of the technical skills that support and save human life.
Specialization is essential to achieving technical competence as
free of error as is humanly possible.

Critical as it is to the healing art, technical skill is limited
in scope and efficacy. Compassionate technicians will ever be
mindful of the degree of human error which, although it cannot be eliminated, can be reduced by sympathetic thorough-
ness. Many examples could be cited, but two will suffice: the
ubiquitous X-rays and laboratory tests.

> A group of three chest specialists and two radiologists col-
> laborated to evaluate the effectiveness of the different sizes
> of X-ray films which had been used by military authorities
> in mass medical examinations of recruits and soldiers. In
> the process of making these comparisons they discovered,
> to their surprise, that they disagreed with each other in
> their interpretations of pathology in about one third of the
> films reviewed, and with themselves when re-examining
> the films, about a fifth of the time. Human factors influenc-
> ing perception and judgment, as opposed to technical ones,
> were found to be the most important causes. The differ-
> ences occurred even though the group beforehand had
> specified the nomenclature they would use in describing
> lesions, and had developed a code for classifying the film
> into categories. Astonished radiologists who reveiwed these
> results and conducted separate trials of their own, con-
> firmed the validity of the findings.[10]

Similar variation in diagnostic results obtains for laboratory tests. The New Jersey Department of Health, having monitored their laboratories since 1963, reported the results to Congress in 1975. Even though laboratories knew they were being monitored, and even though the limits of error established were quite generous, they testified that of 35,000 chemical analyses conducted over a decade by 225 laboratories, only 20 of these 225 laboratories reported acceptable results more than 90 per cent of the time. Half yielded satisfactory results less than 75 per cent of the time, and 9 laboratories less than 50 per cent of the time. Commenting on those results, Dr. Stanley Reiser notes that new techniques of automated laboratory analyses promise to lower such variability, but not eliminate it.[11] Every technique is vulnerable to human and technical error. Compassion requires us to keep human error to a minimum.

But technical medicine is only one expression of our concern for human life. Diagnoses and prognoses are seldom, if ever, purely technical judgments about our capacity to save lives. Judgments are being made constantly about what is worth investigating and who is worth saving. If medicine is to exhibit a genuine respect for persons as living organisms, it will need to be aware of the subtle and not so subtle ways in which persons are not treated as equals.

Another significant boundary on the practice of technical medicine is that its practitioners often have specific views about the meaning of compassion. The very idea of mercy killing suggests that it is sometimes merciful to kill. The judgment that it is or is not merciful to kill is hardly a technical medical judgment. Yet the fate of individual lives will depend upon what view is taken of compassion or mercy.

There is no time in this brief presentation to argue the case against mercy killing.[12] Compassionate medical care does not require it. The usual kinds of exceptions to the injunction not to kill, such as self-defense, seem to have no clear and appropriate analog in medicine—except in abortion to save the life of a pregnant woman. Cicely Saunders, founder of the hospice movement, which has done so much for dying patients, notes her own experience in this regard:

A very small number of patients have wanted to discuss euthanasia with us. No one has come back to make a considered request for us to carry it out. Once pain and the feeling of isolation had been relieved they never asked again.

We had such discussions with two young men, both with motor neuron disease. One said, "If it were available I would ask." Yet he always demanded antibiotics if he had an incipient chest infection and he well knew how inconsistent were his feelings and wishes. Finally he said, "Yes, I would have asked, but now I see the snags." Weighed against all his problems were his deepening relationship with his wife and his growing confidence that we would never let him choke. He died quietly in his sleep after a massive pulmonary embolus. The two of them had shared the hardness throughout and there were no guilts or hang-ups as his wife began her new life.

The other man died later. He found that the stage of physical helplessness in the first, which he had watched with apprehension, was totally different when he reached it himself. He maintained his essential independence, never giving in to anything and fought his way into a peace in which he could say, "I can't see round the next bend but I know it will be all right."[13]

Of course, mercy killing is to be distinguished from our willingness and sometimes our obligation to refrain from various sorts of medical interventions that are neither desired by nor considered in the best interests of persons otherwise presumed to be dying from irreversible conditions. Again, compassion should teach us to respect dying persons as we would others who are living human beings. To care for the dying as persons is surely to care about whether they are lonely and whether they are otherwise occupied in ways that they deem best in their last days. Again, Saunders has beautifully expressed this aspect of care:

A young man said to me, as he faced leaving life and his strong family ties and responsibilities, "I've fought and I've fought—but now I've accepted." We, too, have to learn to accept as well as to fight and to realize that part of our work can have nothing to do with cure but only with the giving of relief and comfort. We will learn by looking at patients, by listening to what they want to say and by meeting their needs as far as we can both practically and philosophically. His readiness finally to say "yes" to death was in itself an affirmation of life. We need him as much and more than he needs us. Anything which says to the very ill or the very old that there is no longer anything that matters in their life would be a deep impoverishment to the whole of society.[14] Another of the boundaries of technical medicine was noted by a medical school dean when he told his graduating class, "Your skills will extend no further than a person's will to live. Any patient who has no will to live will defeat your best efforts." One way in which the will to live is nurtured is by the kind of care that affirms life even in what seem to be bleak physical, psychological or spiritual circumstances. The kind of healing we call faith healing depends on awakening and undergirding that will to live, and extends beyond it to a confidence that healing is available. One context for such confidence is found in our covenant relations, to which we now turn.

Covenant

Sociologist Bernard Barber has recently suggested that compassion in medicine be understood as a form of egalitarian relationship between physicians and patients.[15] He does not dwell on compassion in any of the senses we have already discussed, but focuses entirely on its link with equality. He suggests that medicine needs to train its practitioners to respect patients as equals, as capable of making informed decisions and as bearers of values. He does not claim that physicians and patients can or should be equal in every way, since physicians will bring to the physician-patient relation a type of expertise one cannot expect from patients.

Achievement of a more egalitarian physician-patient relation will certainly depend on cultivating compassion in the form of a willingness to do what is right and an ability to know what is right. Respect for the autonomy and values of patients will need to take the form of recognizing obligations to tell the truth, to keep promises, to honor agreements and to treat people as equals. Without the acceptance of these moral principles and without the willingness to honor them, egalitarianism will be merely an abstract goal, the content of which will be relatively empty and the practice of which will be virtually nil. Thus, for example, I have no quarrel with Barber in insisting on written informed consent that includes the explicit understanding that patients may always break off their relationships with specific physicians; but what it is that patients think they are signing, and the extent to which they feel it is best to comply with physicians, depend very heavily on the integrity, conscientiousness and sympathetic manner of the physicians who seek their consent. The most impeccably written consent forms cannot completely protect patients against those physicians who fail to convey through their words, actions or gestures the true extent of the risks of real pain or loss of life entailed in a therapy or experiment for which consent is being sought.

Hence, although Barber contributes an important insight into one facet of compassion, formal recognition of the liberties and rights of patients will not protect them against the more subtle, often unintentional ways in which physicians obtain from patients what physicians deem best for them. One of the most important protections against mistakes in moral judgment is a genuine sympathy for the condition of the patient, and hence a sensitive awareness of any genuine risks that may be incurred by medical interventions. Similarly, willingness to abide by those moral principles that make possible an appropriate amount of egalitarianism will rest, as we have already indicated, on the extent to which physicians are morally conscientious and morally perceptive.

Respect for human beings as persons, therefore, includes a respect for them as equals. Fundamental to treating others as equals is a complete commitment to truth telling. So often in discussions of truth telling, people ask what harm or benefit will accrue from a contemplated lie, that is, from a contemplated intentional deception. Although it is important to ask that question, and particularly to recognize that lying undermines all human relationships and frustrates cooperative ventures, there is more to lying than that. A lie is depersonalizing. To undertake intentionally to deceive another human being is to treat that human being not as a person but as an object to be manipulated or as an object of one's own unannounced purposes.

However noble the intentions of one who lies, in the act of lying, those intentions are nonnegotiable, and the target of a lie has no defense, no say. In short, the person who is deceived is robbed of the dignity of moral decision making. A moral decision is a choice among perceivable alternatives. What genuine choice is left for those who are misinformed about the true alternatives in a given situation? To lie is to rob persons of their dignity as moral beings. In instances where a patient is in no condition to give consent, truth telling is just as necessary to all the decision makers who genuinely seek to do what is in the patient's best interest.

A covenant between those who wish to heal and those who wish to be healed requires truth telling from everyone in the covenant. Patients who deceive medical professionals frustrate the kind of covenant that makes for healing. Trust is a necessary condition for healing.

Covenants between health professionals and patients are not simply covenants between two individuals. Patients and healers are part of a network of human relations. The family is especially significant. Among the moral bases of a family is the commitment to nurture human life and to express gratitude for the nurture received from parents and the whole community.

Consider the following case. The parents of a child refused to sanction life-saving intervention for their child. Physicians acquiesced to the wishes of the parents. At the time of that decision, children receiving surgery of the kind in question had a life prospect of about twenty years. The parents would not accept that prospect. They saw it as a burdensome and frustrating state of affairs. The irony in this instance is that less than twenty years later, new surgical techniques now guarantee a full life expectancy for children who receive surgery. Some participants in a discussion of this case argued that parents should have the right not to be burdened by children who have a less than full life expectancy. Note how that argument shatters the moral bases of the family. Children are conceived and nurtured, not on the basis of their choosing, but on the basis of commitments made by their parents. Those same parents, like all human beings, are alive because they have been nurtured by others, and because others have chosen not to kill them. Every human community requires that parents be honored. One form of honoring parents is to recognize that life is dependent on the nurture of others and, most immediately, on the sustenance provided by one's own parents. The generosity surrounding the gift of life that each of us enjoys is the least that we can show for others equally at our mercy. That brings us to another aspect of our human existence as persons. We are all part of a larger community.

Community

Whether we acknowledge it or not, it is impossible to be moral if there is no predictable power in us and beyond us to recognize, will and effectuate moral decisions. To claim that it is reasonable to decide for or against an action is to claim, among other things, that we live in a world in which it is possible to believe in our continued existence as human beings and to believe that evil does not always triumph. If it were true that evil would always triumph, why would it be reasonable ever to choose what is right or to choose to prevent or to remove evil —as we constantly do as healers?

There is, then, a kind of healing that technical medicine makes possible, a kind of intervention that sustains our lives as bodies. But as we have observed, technical medicine cannot by itself sustain our bodily existence. We need the assistance of compassionate concern for life and constraints against its devaluation. Human beings also are healed because they are treated with dignity in a covenant of trust, a covenant of truthful exchange of information and concern. Sometimes what happens in such a covenant may be called faith healing.

But now we have come to a third aspect of our being and another kind of healing. We are healed because we have the confidence that we live in a world that is sustained by benign and ultimately triumphant powers. To believe the opposite would make it rational to commit suicide, the ultimate act of rebellion against all healing powers and against the power that sustains life.

The art of healing is often specialized because the various aspects of our being can be separated conceptually—although never completely in actual practice. Taking out an appendix would seem to be a totally technical interchange, but not to persons who despair of life, who will either fail to submit to any treatment or who may even take their lives. By the same token, we can cultivate faith healing because so much of our well-being as human organisms depends on trust and confidence in powerful healing forces that exist within us and around us. Medicine of the whole person would encompass both possibilities, whether in the context of technical medicine or in the context of covenants with persons who claim no technical expertise. Finally, we have created experts of religious faith who encourage confidence in the benign nature of the whole universe. We speak of ministers of the soul. Again, medicine must be open to an aspect of human beings which, if not supported, may thwart any attempt at healing.

The task of medicine is to treat human beings as whole persons, with compassion in a covenant of trust and with an eye to the standards and powers that form, shape and sustain the whole human community. The art of healing requires a love for those standards and powers. We have already talked about a love for the neighbor exhibited in acting in accord with constitutive rules—the rules presupposed in human cooperation. Now we need to consider briefly the kind of guidance available to us in making decisions that strive faithfully to apply these norms in ways that will enhance persons. Where do we find the guidance to be merciful and just?

Consider what we do to obtain justice in our courts. For our purposes, let us imagine the processes used in determining the guilt or innocence of someone who has committed a major crime. The procedures of the court will include the following kinds of processes: (1) fact finding, (2) vividly imagining how it is for the person or persons under consideration by the court and (3) impartiality.

In order to uncover all facts relevant to a case on trial, both a prosecuting and a defense lawyer are necessary. Thus, all facts sympathetic to defending the alleged victim and other potential victims in society are brought out by a prosecutor, and all facts sympathetic to the defendant are brought out by the defendant's lawyer. All of that takes place in the presence of a judge who assures orderly conduct from everyone in the court, so that each person who has information can be heard without interruption or prejudicial commentary.

Increasingly we have come to recognize that the sympathetic portrayal of an alleged victim, on the one hand, and of an alleged perpetrator of a crime, on the other hand, requires more than skilled representation by lawyers. Jurors are expected to imagine how it is for the persons being considered by the court. It is not considered proper to have an all-white jury when a black person is on trial. Similarly, it is not considered appropriate to have an all-male jury when a woman is on trial. We have become aware of subtle influences on our ability to understand how it is for our fellow human beings.

The third standard implicit in the quest of our courts for justice is impartiality. Jurors and judges with obvious biases or conflicts of interest are disqualified from taking part. The use of both defending and prosecuting attorneys is a device explicitly aimed at attending to the diverse and conflicting interests in determining guilt or innocence.

These three standards for rationality in the pursuit of justice are recognized in various philosophical theories.[16] Within the Christian tradition, God has been seen as an ideal moral judge who is omniscient, omnipercipient and totally impartial. God is depicted as both a defending and prosecuting attorney, as one who loves everyone equally, and as one who knows and cares how it is for everyone. From the standpoint of God, all persons have value as his offspring, created in his image. When we are called upon to love God, therefore, we are asked among other things to seek to be knowledgeable, to know how it is for others, and to be impartial in our moral judgments so that, however imperfectly, we may exhibit the mercy and love that are expected of us.

Sometimes in medical writings we find an injunction to use the Golden Rule as a criterion for making moral decisions. It is very helpful to use it as a guideline—that is, to inquire whether we would like to be at the receiving end of any contemplated action. The Golden Rule is not sufficient as a sole guideline, however. It stimulates us to imagine how it is for someone else by imagining how it would be for us, but we must also raise the question of impartiality. A physician, for example, very interested in carrying out some medical research, may be so convinced of the worth of that research that he might be willing to subject himself or others to great risk. I recall an example of that recounted by someone who studied with me. Some fellow physicians were doing research which they described to him. He was astonished at the risks taken in the experiment. They assured him there was no problem because they themselves were serving as the research subjects. But, they were asked, had they consulted their families about this? They had not. It had not occurred to them that members of their own families might express such a concern about their welfare that their participation in the experiments might not have been sanctioned. Their intense interest in the research overshadowed their ability or even willingness to imagine how it was for everyone affected by their actions. They were willing to take such risks, but could they honestly say that others were equally convinced that it was right?

In our sketch of an ethic of the art of healing, we have tried to show in at least a preliminary way the vital roles of compassion and justice. We have also pointed to the necessity to honor certain standards of rationality if compassion and justice are to be served. We have thus restated one of the New Testament summaries of Christian ethics: that we love our neighbors as ourselves, while loving God with all our hearts.

Notes

[1]Raymond S. Duff and A. G. M. Campbell, "Moral and Ethical Dilemmas in the Special-Care Nursery," in *Ethics in Medicine,* ed. Stanley Reiser, Arthur Dyck and William Curran (Cambridge, Mass.: MIT Press, 1977), pp. 539-43.

[2]Ibid.

[3]Joseph Fletcher, "Indicators of Humanhood: A Tentative Profile of Man," *The Hastings Center Report,* 2, No. 5 (Hastings-on-Hudson, N.Y.: Institute of Society, Ethics and the Life Sciences, 1972), 1-4.

[4]Richard A. McCormick, "To Save or Let Die: The Dilemma of Modern Medicine," in *Ethics in Medicine,* pp. 544-48.

[5]Duff and Campbell, p. 541.

[6]"A Right to Die: A Theologian Comments," *Atlantic Monthly,* April 1968, p. 64.

[7]Cited in *Illinois Right to Life Committee Newsletter,* 4, No. 4 (April 1974).

[8]M. Sharon Webb, "Doctors and Dehumanization: Diagnosis and Therapy," unpublished paper.

[9]Ibid., pp. 5-6.

[10]Stanley Joel Reiser, "The Medical Student and the Machine," *Harvard Medical Alumni Bulletin,* 53, No. 1 (September/October 1978), 14.

[11]Ibid., p. 15.

[12]See Arthur J. Dyck, "Living Wills and Mercy Killing: An Ethical Assessment," in *Bioethics and Human Rights: A Reader for Health Professionals,* ed. Bertram and Elsie Bandman (Boston: Little, Brown & Co., 1978), pp. 132-38.

[13]"The Care of the Dying Patient and his Family," in *Ethics in Medicine,* p. 513.

[14]Ibid.

[15]"Compassion in Medicine: Toward New Definitions and New Institutions," *The New England Journal of Medicine,* 295, No. 17 (1976), 939-43.

[16]See Roderick Firth, "Ethical Absolutism and the Ideal Observer," *Philosophy and Phenomenological Research,* XII, No. 3 (March 1952), 317-45; and also William K. Frankena, *Ethics,* 2nd ed. (Englewood Cliffs, N.J.: Prentice-Hall, 1973), pp. 110-14.

Chapter Three

The Tension between Scientific Objectivity and Values in Whole-Person Medicine

Robert L. Herrmann

Within our society strong pressures are often felt to reject science and the objective approach to truth to which it is committed. Good reasons exist for such a reaction, coming from a variety of segments of our culture. Poets have time and again called us back from a too-rigid analysis of human beings and this world. I am especially fond of Elizabeth Barrett Browning, who in her narrative poem "Aurora Leigh" seemed to capture the essence of the material world:

Earth's crammed with heaven,
And every common bush afire with God;
But only he who sees takes off his shoes
The rest sit round it and pluck blackberries... [1]

The same tension has been recognized by many contemporary writers. Commenting on our culture's ambivalent worship of science as material benefactor but spiritual antagonist, Norman Mailer wrote: "there exists at once in us a desire for the most 'objective' scientific facts alongside a yearning to preserve the individual, subjective, and nonscientific view of man and his universe." [2]

The scientific community itself has spawned a few individuals who sense the two-edged nature of science's sword. Speaking at a conference on ethical problems in human genetics, biochemist Leon Kass said:

I suspect that I am not alone among the assembled in considering myself fortunate to be here. For I was conceived after antibiotics yet before amniocentesis, late enough to have benefited from medicine's ability to prevent and control fatal infectious diseases, yet early enough to have escaped from medicine's ability to prevent me from living to suffer from my genetic diseases. To be sure, my genetic vices are, as far as I know them, rather modest, taken individually— myopia, asthma and other allergies, bilateral forefoot adduction, bowleggedness, loquaciousness and pessimism, plus some four to eight as yet undiagnosed recessive lethal genes in the heterozygous condition—but, taken together, and if diagnosable prenatally, I might never have made it.[3]

The present symposium was called partly because many of us sense flaws in the philosophy of scientific objectivity. Our hopes for science have in part been realized in a high material standard of living, remarkable cures of disease and great extraterrestrial feats. Yet at the same time science has been mobilized to build unbelievably destructive weapons and has been misused to foul our water and air. This crisis in values has led to an identity crises which has forced us to plumb the depths of our being. One of the most poignant statements of our predicament comes from naturalist Joseph Wood Krutch, writing on the evolution of man:

If it is really true that he is merely the inevitable culmination of an improbable chemical reaction which happened to take place once and once only and involved "merely material" atoms, then the fact that he has been able to formulate the idea of "an improbable chemical reaction" and to track himself back to it is remarkable indeed. That chemicals which are "merely material" should come to understand their own nature is a staggering supposition. Is it also a preposterous one?

Without attempting to answer that last question one thing more may be said. If it should turn out that man has not understood but misunderstood his own evolution then that is still a fact almost as staggering as understanding it would be. But it is also a staggering irony.

If, to go one step farther, the misunderstanding should lead him to deny, disregard, and allow to atrophy through disuse the very characteristics and powers which most distinguish him—if, in a word, he should thus help himself back down the road he once came up—that would be more than a staggering fact and more than a staggering irony. It would be of all calamities one of the greatest that could befall him—greater perhaps than any except that possibility of falling into the hands of an angry god he once so much feared.[4]

The fantastic picture of "matter" pondering its own origin is for me a worship experience, but my attitude must surely be related to my knowledge of the "angry god."

In that same area of origins, molecular biologist and Nobel Laureate Jacques Monod has written a salient philosophical statement called *Chance and Necessity.*[5] His book presents a totally mechanistic basis for origins, placing man "alone in the unfeeling immensity of the universe," to which he came without meaning and purpose, solely by chance. The compensation for our aloneness, our acceptance of our own contingency, is, Monod says, to be free from "deceitful servitudes" and to be able to "live authentically."

Science as a Spiritual Activity

Underlying the antireligious statements of some scientists is the recurring belief that science arose as an activity competitive with theology—that is, providing an alternative picture of reality. In fact, however, the historical picture is otherwise. Most early scientists were completely at home in God's world. To them the biblical perspective of an utterly trustworthy Creator whose universe was ordered and rational was essential for meaningful experimentation. Albert Einstein much later echoed these sentiments when he referred to a "God who creates and is very difficult to understand, but he is not arbitrary or malicious." As R. Hooykaas pointed out,[6] it is no mistake that our science came out of a Christian culture. In it, to be a scientist was an honorable and worthy occupation, in contrast with the pagan idea of science. For the ancients, nature and the gods who ruled it jealously guarded their secrets from the prying eyes of mortals; Prometheus's theft of the fire could result only in disaster. Biblically, the picture is quite different. As Donald MacKay explained in a superb discussion of biblical perspectives on human engineering:

> The Bible sets man in perspective as a creature of God, a part of the vast created order that owes its continuance in being to the divine upholding power. Unlike the rest of the natural world known to us, however, human beings have powers of foresight, planning and action that make us specially responsible in the eyes of our Creator. With these powers, according to the Bible, goes a special obligation toward the Creator. Men are commanded, not merely permitted, to "subdue the earth" (Gen. 1:28). This is not to be done, indeed, in a spirit of arrogant independence, but as the stewards of God's creation.
>
> Human beings are answerable to Him for the effectiveness with which they have fulfilled His mandate. Our overriding priority from the biblical standpoint is to love God and our neighbor. All human exploitation of natural laws and resources must be an expression of this love, and of nothing else, if it is to be acceptable.
>
> The Christian ethos is in complete contrast to the pagan caricature with which it is so often confused. In place of craven fear that haunts the unwelcome interloper, we are meant to enjoy the peaceful confidence of a servant-son at home in his Father's creation. We know that we are on our Father's business no less when investigating His handiwork than when engaged in formal acts of worship. In place of jealously secretive gods we have One whose very nature is Truth, and Light, Himself the giver of all that is true, who rejoices when any of His truth is brought to the light and obeyed in humility.[7]

So the scientist is no unwelcome interloper but a servant-son in his Father's creation. As the Oxford physicist Charles Coulson once said, the practice of science is to be seen as a fit activity for a Sabbath afternoon.[8]

Science, in return, has given the theologian a real world. As Walter Thorson expressed it, "medieval society and medieval thought were . . . centered on a fundamentally religious conceptual framework with a papier-mâché sort of physical universe which had no more meaning than a kind of 'stage prop' on which the drama of salvation was enacted."[9] By comparison, science "took the secular world and the secular calling more seriously. Instead of a papier-mâché universe, God had made a real one, and the basic inspiration for the scientific revolution was a passionate belief that, in exploring and knowing what God had given us men in creation, we would find a larger framework in which our grasp of our role and destiny—could grow and develop further."

The challenge came in the words of Francis Bacon, "if . . . there be any humility towards the Creator, if there be any reverence for or disposition to magnify His works, if there be any charity for man . . . we should approach with humility and veneration to unroll the volume of Creation."[10] Science thus came as an outgrowth of religious concern, not as a competitor but rather as a complementary activity, to enlarge our view of God's creation.

Complementary Views of Reality

The idea of complementary views of reality was once described in an analogy by physicist Charles Coulson. During World War 2 he was responsible for building a new physics laboratory at the University of London. Because of space limitations and because of the bombing, it was decided to build the laboratory beneath the quadrangle. On occasion, Coulson met with the architects and reviewed plans for that unseen building. He studied the various drawings and blueprints: floor plans, sections, elevations—some detailed, some rough. None was complete, none exhaustive, though each was complete in itself.

Professor Coulson saw in those plans an apt analogy to the nature of truth. The various drawings were like the different disciplines: science, history, the Scriptures, music, art (and, being an Englishman, he added poetry). Thus there were many descriptions of reality, the unseen building, but none was complete or exhaustive or exclusive.

As another example we might consider a rose. The poet says, "A rose is a rose is a rose." The theologian might say, "A rose is God's herald of summer." The scientist might say, "A rose is that part of the rose plant that bears the reproductive apparatus: stamens, pistil, petals and so forth." Each gives a valid description of a rose, but each says something different. With such a view of reality, the idea of exclusiveness of knowledge in any one discipline disappears. All have some part in describing unseen reality.

In that context, scientific objectivity (as usually defined) takes on the appearance of arrogant exclusivism. Its definition, as supplied by the philosophical structure of logical positivism, specifies that:

1. Only scientific statements are valid.

2. Scientific statements are impersonal.

3. Only scientific method is valid as a means to discover truth.

4. Personal choices, subjective experiences, states of mind and so on are intrinsically meaningless.

Continued acceptance of the exclusive "objectivist" position by significant numbers of medical faculty bodes ill for the prospect of producing whole-person physicians. Can a patient expect to be regarded as having more significance than a disease if it is implicit in the diagnosis that only scientifically measurable quantities are meaningful? As we shall see, however, the objectivist position is not a necessary consequence of a rigorous scientific posture.

Some years ago I read an article in a Boston area Christian newspaper called the *Cambridge Fish*.[11] The article, with the rather heavy title "The Concept of Truth in the Natural Sciences," was written by a friend of mine at MIT, Professor Walter Thorson, who was mentioned earlier. He was introducing his readers to some important new concepts of truth developed by physicist-turned-philosopher Michael Polanyi, an eminent British scientist with experience in both physical and behavioral sciences who was then at the University of

Manchester. The essence of Polanyi's work was to show that the search for scientific truth does not have the infallible, impersonal objectivity generally attributed to it, but that unavoidable nonobjective components in science have a significant bearing on our truth seeking.[12]

It is granted that objective evaluation is an essential ingredient in science, and that our data owe much of their validity to the extent to which we can avoid our own biases as we gather them. But Polanyi points out that there are, in fact, tacit presuppositions which we bring to bear in our evaluation of the data, as we construct our hypotheses. Words like *simple, beautiful, satisfying, fruitful* are used, which say more than they should if we are in fact totally objective in articulating our theory. Thorson explains the results of Polanyi's historical study of the motivations of scientific discovery and scientific theorizing this way:

> It is standard logical positivist dogma to assert that scientific theories are merely logical orderings of empirical facts in the most economical fashion. Polanyi shows that many major theoretical achievements have been made as the outcome of a heuristic search for rational beauty, satisfying the intellectual passions of the searcher; this recognition of beauty is accepted and accredited by the searcher and by his trained peers as a guide to the structure of reality which is as important as the process of empirical validation to the achievements of science. According to logical positivism we can have no basis for choosing between two theories if both give an economical description of the same empirical facts. Professor Polanyi asserts that such an attitude is incorrect; in reality, a scientist assesses a theory not only for its empirical validity but also for its rational appeal to him personally and for its capacity to evoke a larger conception of reality as a whole, of which the previously known is but a part. This is not to ignore the necessity of empirical observation by any means, but to show the absurdity of the positivist claim that the appreciation of rational excellence plays no essential role in scientific discovery.[13]

The exciting conclusion of this analysis is that even scientific truth gathering requires personal commitment; it requires, in Polanyi's words, "a passionate contribution in the personal act of knowing." And, in case we have not made the connection to another kind of Truth gathering, Polanyi closes his treatise with the words, "And that is also, I believe, how a Christian is placed when worshipping God."

We see, then, that scientific truth gathering is not, *nor can it be,* the totally objective, exclusive source of truth which Jacques Monod purported it to be. We intuitively introduce value components into our hypothesizing, and not only is that unavoidable, but it actually *helps* us to arrive at the correct hypothesis. It is tempting to say, in present company, that we have discovered that a "whole person" will perform the best scientific thinking.

An additional point relating wholeness to truth gathering should be considered. The major competitor of objectivism among philosophical theories is existentialism. Existentialism is an example of exclusivism in the opposite direction—again a violation of the principle of complementary ways of knowing, and a denial, I think, of personal wholeness. Modern existentialist philosophy states that our subjective feelings and attitudes are self-authenticating, regardless of the availability of an external reality structure to which those feelings and attitudes refer. The extreme example which recurs often in our culture is the statement, "It doesn't matter what you believe, as long as you believe it sincerely." Existentialist thought has had great impact on our religious institutions. Modern existentialist theology asserts that biblical statements receive meaning as a function of their impact on an individual; that is, I give meaning to what I read by whether I react to it or not. In the vernacular it might be said, "If it turns me on, it has meaning." Thorson's critique of existentialism includes a discussion of the nature of truth as follows:

> When we speak of the truth, we imply that we are responsible to it as something we did not create for ourselves, but something we *discovered.* We are obligated to think in the framework we call the truth, and to expect continuity and

consistency; the truth is not a function of our state of mind but evokes responsibility in our state of mind. This emphasis on responsibility and continuity in our approach to reality, totally obvious in matters scientific, is a crucial reference point when we consider the pure subjectivity propounded as reality by extreme forms of existentialism. We are bound not only to share our perception of reality with other knowers, but to be bound by it ourselves, as an interpretive framework for experience. Extreme existentialism rejects this obligation on the ground that it is a restriction of freedom, but if we look at the scientific achievements gained by the disciplined truth of science, we can see how silly this is. Life is not to be approached in an unstructured fashion, moving from one raw experience to another; such a procedure amounts to the denial of truth altogether and is a refusal to be affected by it. Extreme existentialism's radical negation of objective, consistent structure in the world must be rejected if we wish to keep faith with the concept of reality we encounter in science, for example. The existential reality of self cannot be dissociated from the consistent setting in which it is placed. We are, but there is also that which is not us, and is both real and true. We are responsible to try to see it correctly.

The emphasis of existentialism on a cleavage with the world of objectivity, consistency and structure is at least in part a reaction against the positivist epistemology. A theory of the world in which man himself is confidently reduced to mere mechanistic processes, analyzed biologically, psychologically and sociologically, and in the process deprived of his existential freedom by this analysis, is indeed a terrifying prospect, and no sensitive human being could really tolerate it, even if it were true. Perhaps the determination of many existentialists to maintain a complete philosophical discontinuity with the world where structure, mechanism and consistency exist is the result of secret ambivalence toward the positivist world-view; they are afraid it is really true.[14]

Thus, we may conclude that these two mutually exclusive views of reality, objectivism and extreme existentialism, have been destructive of both science and theology. In science they have led to a depersonalization of the truth seeker with a consequent disregard of the ethical dimension in the application of scientific truth. In theology they have allowed man to be torn out of his biblical role as the God-breathed, responsible servant-son in his Father's creation and to be enthroned as his own ultimate authority without reference point or direction. As Paul Tillich has said, "We live in a land of broken symbols." By comparison, the biblical position is that all truth and authority come from God as the great Revealer; the truth we learn through the scientific enterprise and the truth that comes through faith in Jesus Christ form part of one "given" fabric of reality. At just this point a true view of scientific objectivity comes to our support as believers in the historic Christian faith. I believe we have the utmost to gain by recognition of the essentiality of objective data lying outside ourselves and referring to some external reality—because we have verified documentation in the form of the Scriptures as a unique data base in Christianity. Again the complementary character of truth reveals its importance. The effectiveness of the scientific method warns us away from too subjective a view of faith and helps us to be faithful to the biblical revelation.

Negative Consequences of Exclusive Views of Truth
The practical consequences of objectivism and extreme existentialism have been devastating to ourselves and our cultural institutions. Modern existentialist theology has been the avenue of invasion for various forms of mysticism and, most important, has produced what is commonly referred to as the "cool culture." For large numbers of people, particularly those in their late adolescence and their early twenties, reality is only immediate, unplanned and unreflected experience. They have become ready partakers of certain techniques of Far Eastern religions, the "incense-burners and inner spacemen," as Thorson refers to them.[15]

The pervasive nature of their thought pattern is difficult to describe adequately. It doubtless affects a large percentage of undergraduates preparing for medical school. As a biochemistry professor, I would like to think that it is also part of the reason medical and dental students manage so effectively to subdue enthusiasm for my discipline. I recall a chemistry professor at MIT once telling me that a freshman had come up to him after a lecture on the periodic table with the serious question, "You don't really believe that, do you?"

Such pure subjectivism has introduced into the holistic medicine movement a number of Eastern religious techniques. Among them are use of various mind-altering drugs and incense, yoga, transcendental meditation and Zen. In spite of sporadic efforts to provide an objective basis for transcendental meditation and Zen, the overall indictment must be made that such techniques have no rational basis derivable from verifiable objective data. They relate clearly to no external reality structure. I therefore set these categories aside as both qualitatively and quantitatively different from the prayer of faith which has as its object the healing which comes from the God of the Bible.

Let us examine one additional practical problem foisted on us by an exclusivist view—this time the effect of objectivism on the kind of thinking that scientists and health professionals are capable of when confronted with ethical problems. One of the reasons I left Boston to help start the new medical school at Oral Roberts was my conviction that there was a crisis of integrity in medicine. I considered it to be of such proportions that only a bold stroke of departure from the norm would be effective.

Through a friend on the Boston University publications staff, I was asked to write an article for the university newspaper which called for a return to religious values, preferably biblical values, in the preparation of premedical students, selection of students for admission to medical school and the preparation of the medical-school curriculum.[16] What struck me was the almost total lack of concern for ethics on the part of educators in the face of phenomenal growth of technical advances in the medical sciences and the corresponding enormity of ethical problems they pose. At a 1976 symposium on recombinant DNA technology, psychologist Gerald Holton stated that fewer than one per cent of scientists indicate any interest in ethics.[17] Molecular biologist Robert Sinsheimer, who spoke at the Human Engineering Conference at Wheaton several years ago, said that at Cal Tech he was alone in his interest and burden for bioethics.[18] Jacques Monod's view of the dangers of genetic engineering is that they are "an illusion, spread by a few superficial minds."[19]

Despite the establishment of many new ethics courses in recent years, it is still not clear that human values are a priority in medical education. In light of the incredibly large disparity between the problem and the means to a solution, I am convinced that the value systems of our physicians and other health professionals must be developed much earlier, with a strong foundation in the Judeo-Christian tradition.[20] I make no excuse for this bias. It is clear, as even outspoken foes of Christianity like Monod have admitted, that our culture functions with either explicit or implicit adherence to Judeo-Christian values. Humanism has no alternatives to offer, as Os Guinness demonstrated in *The Dust of Death*.[21] In view of the paucity of other value systems, I propose that we call for a re-examination of the roots of our religious tradition as part of the education of every health professional. That should motivate Christian educators to direct their best efforts toward producing course materials in medical ethics suitable for the secular universities. It should also encourage the various religiously oriented high schools and colleges to upgrade their science and philosophy programs.

The few dozen Christian colleges now providing serious preprofessional preparation should expand their programs. The number of such schools should be multiplied in order to contribute a higher proportion of biomedical scientists and health professionals. Beyond that, what is developing at Oral Roberts University may provide a new model for integrated learning (see pp. 16-17).

Toward an Integration of Medicine and Prayer

Whole-person medicine seems to provide an ideal structure within which to trace a middle course between the extremes of objectivism and pure subjective experience. I submit that both the biblical revelation of God, and the science which the Bible has nurtured and which should be seen as a complementary view of reality, form crucial elements for our understanding of our existence and of our health. Human health must take into account the multifaceted nature of a tripartite being made in the image of God. The equation for healing therefore must contain elements of physical, psychological, cultural and spiritual character, each factor properly weighted by its reference to the biblical perspective of human meaning and purpose.

When the Medical Ethics Commission of the Christian Medical Society met to plan this conference some two years ago, there began a dialog on "faith healing" which revealed an interesting diversity of opinion among the commission members. Two of them produced a proposal for circulation to the rest, the elements of which are essentially as follows: Man as God's creation is said to possess a nature that is both spiritual and physical. His spiritual nature is viewed as "supernatural" and his physical nature as part of a "natural" category. God's desire for man's wholeness is realized ordinarily by natural means through his divine creation and infrequently by supernatural means through his divine grace. "Natural healing," is achieved by the "rational application of the natural laws of God's creation." "Supernatural healing" is achieved through "divine grace usually applied in response to prayer made in the name of Jesus Christ and for his glory."

In my opinion that statement is inadequate for several reasons. First, the categories *natural* and *supernatural* provoke an unbiblical view of the separation of the physical and the spiritual. The thrust of the statement is that physical healing is normative, usual and derives from the way God originally created man. It leaves out the whole sweep of biblical teaching concerning God's immanent activity in sustaining his creation, an emphasis beautifully described by Donald MacKay.

MacKay notes that a view of God as a kind of machine-tender still lingers in our thinking. The world is seen as a great machine which God created and from which he then largely withdrew except for rare interferences called miracles. Yet MacKay points out that:

> The Bible as a whole represents God in far too intimate and active a relationship to daily events to be represented in these mechanical terms. He does not come in only at the beginning of time to "wind up the works"; he continually "upholds all things by the word of His power" (Hebrews 1:3). "In Him [that is, Christ] all things hold together" (Colossians 1:17).
>
> Here is an idea radically different from that of tending or interfering with a machine. It is not only the physically inexplicable happenings (if any) but the whole going concern that the Bible associates with the constant activity of God.[22]

In that view, God is as active in the efficacy of a drug as he is in the answer to a prayer for healing, so we should not deprive him of the first category by calling it the "rational application of the natural laws of his creation." The use of *natural* and *supernatural* also leads to confusion when viewed from the human side. George Engel has noted that at a recent Rockefeller Foundation seminar on the concept of health, one authority urged that medicine "concentrate on the 'real diseases' and not get lost in the psychosociological under-brush. The physician should not be saddled with problems that have arisen from the abdication of the theologian and the philosopher."[23] The implication of that and other remarks was that the "real" or "organic elements" of disease were the tangible or natural ones which the physician could handle; God and the theologians or any other takers could have the rest.

Engel then went on to point out that the biomedical model had its roots in the historic controversy of the Renaissance church over mind-body dualism in which religious authority allowed study of the human body but included a "tacit interdiction against corresponding investigation of man's mind and behavior. With such a mind-body dualism firmly established under the imprimatur of the church, classical science readily fostered the notion of the body as a machine, of disease as the consequence of breakdown of the machine, and of the doctor's task as repair of the machine."[24]

As Engel asserted, the biomedical model has been enormously successful, but at a cost. What we are seeing in our society is the beginning of a recognition that health is a composite of physical, environmental, emotional, sociological and spiritual factors which form a unique matrix for each patient. To ignore all but the first entity because the other factors are less tangible or are obscured by the "underbrush" is unrealistic for medical professionals.

Again, some of the difficulty is surely attributable to the exclusivism of the objectivist position. We must constantly remind ourselves that there are valid descriptions of reality other than the scientific one. Further, such descriptions, though they often assault our penchant for precision and focus, are probably rather accurate considering the complexity of all the factors. A similar plea was entered by anthropologist Margaret Mead in her 1976 presidential address to the American Association for the Advancement of Science, "Towards a Human Science." After expressing concern that we avoid "inappropriate extension into the physical world of human beings' understanding of themselves," thus signaling her allegiance to scientific objectivity, Mead went on to suggest that "the extension into the human world of the methods of the physical sciences can be stultifying and dangerous. It is only when we do recognize that there are two distinct complementary—rather than antagonistic—sources of knowledge that we can fully develop methods appropriate to each and consider how such methods can serve to support and reinforce each other."[25]

Human and Divine Agency

Finally, we need to examine the biblical relationship between human and divine agency. Scripture does not delineate spheres or zones of activity for God and man. The apostle

Paul wrote, "Work out your own salvation with fear and trembling; for God is at work in you, both to will and to work for his good pleasure" (Phil. 2:12-13). The saying, "Work as though all depended on you; pray as though all depended on God," comes close to the mark. The agency of God is not an alternative to that of his creatures but rather a necessary condition of the agency of his creatures. That is true regardless of whether the focus is on his role as Creator or as Redeemer. As Creator, not only has he brought the universe into being, but he upholds it; he maintains it in continuance (Heb. 1:3). To uphold it is to hold it in being by his power. The question is not one of our action apart from God, because apart from his "holding in being" there would be nothing. We would cease to exist. But we know also that God is related to us personally, as father to son, and so as his creatures our relationship to him is that of a servant-son at home in his Father's creation.

We do not "wrest from Nature her secrets"; rather we are given truth about creation by God with the expectation that we will act in responsible freedom. The responsibility is not to be taken lightly. "We are," as Donald MacKay has put it, "feeling our way to the controls of a world whose mechanism is unimaginably more complex and delicately balanced than we are ever likely to comprehend."[26] If we are to act responsibly then "we shall need a wisdom infinitely greater than our own," and we should take courage in the promise of Scripture that if we lack wisdom we may "ask God, who gives to all men generously and without reproaching" (Jas. 1:5).

Over the last few years I have grown in appreciation for God's provision of wisdom for the truth seeker through the Holy Spirit. I have been especially impressed with Jesus' words in John 16 where he promises "the Comforter" (v. 7 KJV) and then elaborates on his function: "when the Spirit of truth comes, he will guide you into all the truth" (v. 13). Arthur Holmes describes the standard Christian position on the Spirit's function in truth gathering. He excludes John 16 from any relevance to "scientific or philosophical beliefs" and goes on to say that with reference to those categories the

Spirit's work is a mind-clearing and thought-focusing activity that "helps us get things in clearer relationship to the essential content of the Christian faith." Finally, Holmes says that the difference the Holy Spirit makes is not that we as scientists have private sources of information or become better thinkers, but that our "final rule of faith and practice is clearly identified as the Scriptures, and the focus of [our] thinking the ultimate unity of truth: Jesus Christ as creator and lord."[27]

It is precisely at that point, at the understanding of Jesus Christ as Creator and Lord, that I begin to re-examine the Holy Spirit's role. If the Spirit is to guide us into all the truth about Jesus Christ, then should we not expect to perceive better the creation he has made? Shouldn't the restoration of the communion which Adam had with his Father be expected to bring with it some vestige of the remarkable wisdom Adam must have had as he named the animals (Gen. 2:19) and as he fulfilled his responsibility to "till [the garden of Eden] and keep it" (Gen. 2:15)? And in the present context, should we not ask whether as whole-person scientists and whole-person physicians we are utilizing spiritual resources adequately?

Should not the Spirit of God be as active as we "open the volume of creation" as when we open the Scriptures? The approach to answers to such questions excites me. As a member of a growing Christian community of medical scientists (some three dozen at present), I believe new ground may be broken here in understanding God's truth. Already we meet together to pray for our research. As the patients come and as the clinical faculty grows, we see opportunity for new dimensions of cooperation in understanding and enhancing the healing process.

All this seems appropriate when we think back to the complementary nature of divine and human agency. If God's activity is a necessary condition of ours, then should we not expect, as those indwelt by his Spirit, to experience his help as we design our experiments or as we integrate a patient's various indications in arriving at a diagnosis? There is tremendous potential here to bring the whole sweep of human experience—whether through the more objective approach of the physical sciences or the more subjective avenues of religion and the arts—into dynamic relationship to the sovereign God, recognizing finally that "the whole multi-patterned drama of the universe is His."[28]

Notes

[1]*The Complete Poetical Works of Elizabeth Barrett Browning*, Book VII (Boston: Houghton Mifflin, 1900).

[2]*Of a Fire on the Moon* (New York: Signet, 1971).

[3]"Implications of Prenatal Diagnosis for the Human Right of Life," in *Ethical Problems in Human Genetics*, ed. Hilton et al. (New York: Plenum, 1973), pp. 185-99.

[4]*The Great Chain of Life* (New York: Pyramid Books, 1956), p. 171.

[5]Jacques Monod, *Chance and Necessity* (New York: Vintage Books, 1972).

[6]R. Hooykaas, *Christian Faith and the Freedom of Science*, Philosophia Lebera (London: Tyndale Press, 1957).

[7]Donald MacKay, "Biblical Perspectives on Human Engineering," in *Modifying Man: Implications and Ethics*, ed. C. W. Ellison (Washington, D.C.: University Press of America, 1977), pp. 68-69.

[8]*Science and Christian Belief* (Oxford: Oxford University Press, 1954).

[9]Walter Thorson, "The Christian and the Sciences," Century 3 Lecture, Grace Chapel, Lexington, Mass., 1975.

[10]Hooykaas, p. 18.

[11]Walter Thorson, "The Concept of Truth in the Natural Sciences," *Themelios*, 5 (1968), 27-39; rpt. in *Cambridge Fish*, 3, No. 3.

[12]*Personal Knowledge* (New York: Harper Torchbooks, 1964).

[13]Thorson, "The Concept of Truth in the Natural Sciences."

[14]Ibid.

[15]Walter Thorson, "The Spiritual Dimensions of Science," in *Horizons in Science: Christian Scholars Speak Out*, ed. C. F. Henry (New York: Harper & Row, 1978), pp. 217-57.

[16]Donald Clark, "The Crisis of Integrity in Medicine," *Spectrum*, 3, No. 9 (Boston: Boston University Publications, 1976), 4-5.

[17]"Scientific Optimism and Societal Concerns," *Annals of the New York Academy of Science*, 265 (1976), 82-101.

[18]"Genetic Intervention and Values," in Ellison, *Modifying Man*, pp. 109-26.

[19]Monod, p. 17.

[20]Robert Herrmann, "The Recombinant DNA Controversy: Could Anything But Good Come Out?" *Journal of the American Scientific Affiliation*, 30 (1978), 73-74. See also Herrmann, "Molecular Biology in the Dock," in Henry, *Horizons in Science*, pp. 117-29.

[21]*The Dust of Death* (Downers Grove, Ill.: InterVarsity Press, 1973).

[22]Donald MacKay, *Science and Christian Faith Today* (London: CPAS Publications, 1973), p. 10. See also *The Clockwork Image* (Downers Grove, Ill.: InterVarsity Press, 1974).

[23]"The Need for a New Medical Model: A Challenge for Biomedicine," *Science,* 196 (1977), 129-36.

[24]Ibid.

[25]"Towards a Human Science," *Science,* 191 (1976), 903-9.

[26]MacKay, "Biblical Perspectives on Human Engineering."

[27]*All Truth Is God's Truth* (Grand Rapids, Mich.: Eerdmans, 1977), pp. 122-23.

[28]MacKay, *Science and Christian Faith Today.*

Part II

Medical Education

Chapter Four

Whole-Person Medicine and Scientific Medicine

John R. Brobeck

Since the stated purpose of this symposium is to "define whole-person medicine and establish goals that will become the foundation for meaningful programs," I shall try to move toward that goal (1) by reviewing where medicine and medical education have been during the past fifty years and where we are now and (2) by suggesting how our recent history may be used in the development of a whole-person concept of medical practice. To do that it will be necessary to note some of the problems that must be faced if whole-person medicine is to be introduced into the medical curriculum as a philosophy of medical education as well as of medical practice.

I used the phrase *scientific medicine* in my title because many persons suppose that whole-person medicine is in competition or even in conflict with scientific medicine. Thus, after my name appeared on the program of this meeting, I received a letter from a former medical student. He wrote that he recalled well our course in physiology and therefore was surprised to see my name listed here. He remembered the strong experimental emphasis of our course and he judged that emphasis to be at variance with the aims of this symposium. In my reply I assured him that I have not given up my interest in education for scientific medicine.

Historical Perspective

One should recall that for the past hundred years, that is, since about 1880, medical education in this country has followed a course charted by President Charles W. Eliot of Harvard, by Mr. Johns Hopkins and by the persons to whom Johns Hopkins entrusted the founding of a university, a hospital and a medical school. Abraham Flexner's famous report did not appear until some thirty years later (1910).[1] By that time the Johns Hopkins School of Medicine (and, to a lesser degree, Harvard) had set standards against which Flexner could measure all the schools of the U.S. and Canada. He was not the one, therefore, who originated the concept of a university-based, scientifically oriented medical curriculum for American Schools. It was he, however, who brought public opinion to bear on the disgraceful conditions he found during his survey. No doubt Flexner's greatest achievement was the enlisting of the support of the John D. Rockefellers, senior and junior, who with the resources of the General Education Board financed the creation of a handful of other first-rate medical schools across the country.[2]

Flexner ended one chapter of his 1910 report with these words: "One closes a brief review of the medical sciences with a feeling akin to dismay. So much remains to find out, so much is already known,—how futile to orient the student from either standpoint! Practically, however, there is no ground for despair. Enough can be achieved to give him precise conceptions in each of the realms touched upon. . . . After a strenuous laboratory discipline the student will still be ignorant of many things, but at any rate he will respect facts: he will have learned how to obtain them, and what to do with them when he has them."[3]

To decide whether or not the scientific revolution in medical education was successful, and whether it has been completed, it is necessary to know what its goals were. They can be stated most easily in the form of negatives—the qualities that Flexner associated with inferior medical education. Essentially there were four deficiencies, as follows: (1) substandard schools had no relations with a university or merely nominal relations with a parent university; (2) standards for admission were lax and not enforced; (3) teaching was didactic, by lecture only; and (4) there was no laboratory experience or only token laboratory work.

Seventy years after Flexner began his study, one can see that even now his first criterion has not been met universally in American medical education. Thus in many medical schools the university relationship he called for is little more than an administrative supervision by a remote parent. In other instances the creation of a "medical university" having schools of medicine, nursing, allied medical professions, pharmacy, dentistry and a graduate program in medical sciences is taken to be the equivalent of a university connection.

Neither of these conditions is the ideal Flexner had in mind. Yet probably they are as effective as those in the two schools Flexner used for his comparison, where a geographical separation of medicine from the rest of the university is of long-standing duration. Oral Roberts University has in this regard an opportunity lacking in many other medical centers, because here the school of medicine is located in the midst of the university.

As to the second criterion, at present there is little criticism of admissions standards. They may be higher than Flexner anticipated. Occasionally one does see a question as to whether the intense competition that exists for places in medical classes may not be a deterrent to the best kind of college preparation for medicine. Less stress on science and a broader interest in humanities are recommended, as they have been for at least the past forty years. Such recommendations are said to be ineffective, however, because college students are convinced that admissions committees are interested mainly in what has been accomplished in science courses.

As a matter of fact and of record, faculties of basic science departments are not recommending that students major in science, and especially not in biology or psychology. We are satisfied if a student has had only a single modern course in biology, provided that he or she is soundly grounded in modern chemistry and physics and is capable of facing an algebraic equation without feeling faint. In place of the ability to use logarithms and a slide rule, familiarity with a "scientific" model pocket calculator is now sufficient.

With reference to the third and fourth criteria, namely, teaching methods and laboratory instruction, there is some cause for concern. Many teachers of medical science are disturbed because laboratory experience in their courses has become a casualty of two attacks: student protests against time spent in laboratories and revised curricula that shorten the hours given to basic science courses. In general, the more aggressive the students and the more progressive the curriculum, the less the laboratory instruction.

Nevertheless, with that loss there has come a major gain, in that the didactic form of teaching—that is, lectures to be memorized—has practically disappeared in the clinical disciplines. Moreover, even in the science courses the time given to didactic instruction has not been increased. If anything, it too has been shortened, because as the laboratories have been dropped the time thereby freed has not been diverted to lectures. It is given, rather, to small-group conferences.

It would be interesting to be able to compare quantitatively the effectiveness of teaching science in a lecture-laboratory format with that of the lecture-conference plan. I suppose that everyone who taught basic medical science courses under the curricula of twenty years ago remembers that our students were not enchanted with what we were trying to do. Rather, many students resented both us and our courses and carried that resentment through all the years of their professional life. The science courses were regarded as rites of initiation or even as hazing, which prospective doctors had to undergo. That being the case, one can argue that students may leave the contemporary lecture-conference courses with a less hostile attitude toward scientists and science and therefore be more receptive to the concept of scientific medical practice than were students of a generation earlier.

One additional feature of a progressive curriculum should be mentioned. Although there is a tendency to evaluate a curriculum mainly for what it offers to future practitioners, it is equally important to assess how effective it is in recruiting and training the next generation of medical investigators. It is essential to maintain in medical schools the open doors that lead to proficiency in science, at least for some students, such as those who will make their careers in biomedical science or in clinical research and teaching. A curriculum designed so that as a minimum it meets the needs of those students who eventually will become practitioners, may at the same time offer more opportunity in science than did the older, traditional plans. Elective time can be spent in scientific training at an advanced level. A student interested in biochemistry, for example, may be able to take courses usually offered only to graduate students and may be able also to spend time in a research laboratory. That can be of utmost significance to an important fraction of every medical class.

The Incomplete Revolution in Scientific Medicine
Both in education and in practice, therefore, medicine has been undergoing a scientific revolution for nearly a hundred years. But it is a revolution that is not complete and probably never will be completed. I believe it is unfair to say that the scientific model of medical care has failed. On the contrary, we have yet to learn how to make it work.

We still graduate hundreds of students who are not capable of using and who do not want to use, scientific methods in their practice. That statement does not refer to laboratory gadgets and tests. It refers, rather, to the following:

1. In the scientific practice of medicine, the sequence begins with taking a patient's history and progresses through physical examination, a tentative diagnosis, and laboratory and other examinations, to diagnosis and therapy. Such a sequence should be consciously recognized as the analog of the scientific sequence of data gathering, hypothesis, experiment and thesis. To practice with full benefit of a scientific perspective, a doctor should recognize the steps in the process, know just where the study of a particular patient stands at any given moment, and know where to backtrack when predic-

tions or expectations do not come to pass.

2. A physician should know how to systematize the collection of results from a medical practice and how to arrive at reliable conclusions, so that his or her understanding and skill may improve from personal experience.

3. Every physician should know how to evaluate published results, including the strategy, planning, execution and data presented, so that professional growth and education may continue on the basis of the wealth of literature available for that purpose.

If all medical students left school with such capabilities and with an ambition to use them, there would be little need for legal requirements for continuing medical education and re-licensure. The need to familiarize all medical students with the scientific method is just as important now as it was years ago. Medical education has a long way to go before it can say it has attained that objective.

For that reason one must ask the question, "How many objectives can a medical school aim for?" If a school should adopt as a goal the teaching of whole-person medicine, would it be obliged to relax its attention to scientific medicine? No one knows the answer. We do know, however, that at the present time no medical faculty is working unanimously toward a single objective. In the face of strong forces impelling schools toward a scientific orientation, other points of view can be discerned in medical (especially clinical) departments. Very often the philosophies of educational objections have been layered like a chocolate cake. Teachers of medical sciences have planned their courses as if science were the only proper goal, and students have had to submit to that philosophy whether they like it or not. When they attained their third and fourth years, many of them decided that they had not liked it, and soon discovered that many members of the clinical faculty were not really at home in science, either. With the new curricula the situation has changed only in that the philosophies are no longer stratified; they are oriented in parallel. Students can thereby better compare them, and perhaps draw upon the virtues of each.

At the same time another change has taken place. At least in the stronger schools the clinical departments often include at least a few teachers well trained in science, interested in research and able to carry on active experimental programs in their own laboratories. (They are the ones who are criticized because they are said to be hardly ever available for consultations.) This brings to the attention of students the fact that science and medicine do not have to be separated, and demonstrates how clinicians can be also investigators. I am told, however, that because of inadequate attention to science in medical schools and in postgraduate education the number of well-qualified clinical investigators in this country is actually decreasing at the present time.

In view of the problems that conflicting philosophies may create in a school's curriculum, one must ask just how the whole-person concept will be introduced. For example, will biochemists, microbiologists and anatomists be expected to find a way to direct their courses toward such a goal? Can we avoid the preparation of another kind of layer cake, with science mainly in the first year or so, and whole-person medicine reserved for the clinics, wards and clinical electives? It will be of first importance not to permit the faculty to divide itself into those interested in science and those interested in whole-person medicine, as faculties traditionally are divided into scientists and physicians.

In preparing for this conference I read an account of the epidemics of smallpox that invaded Boston and Philadelphia in the early eighteenth century. At that time variolation was available as an effective, although not ideal, preventive, but was largely unused. If I had been a colonial physician in Boston in 1712, would I have applied myself to caring for as many as possible of the 6,000 persons ravaged by the disease? Or would I have tried systematically to evaluate the efficacy of variolation? In fact, Cotton Mather and a certain Dr. Zabdiel Boylston did encourage variolation at the time of that epidemic. Nevertheless, forty years later, in 1752, Boston suffered another epidemic in which nearly 8,000 persons out of a population of nearly 16,000 had the disease, and 539 died.[4]

It is important to consider that historical situation in a personal way and to try to imagine what we might have done, because to a degree all of us are making similar choices now. Do we give ourselves to the care of patients with poliomyelitis, or do we develop a vaccine? Do we care for patients with terminal renal disease or learn what causes it and how to prevent it? Develop more new operations for restoring blood flow or search for causes of hypertension and atherosclerosis? I have no hesitation in saying that the response of this audience to these questions will be an emphatic "Both." We must be careful, therefore, in all planning for medical education to preserve and even strengthen the opportunities for training in both directions.

An interesting sidelight on these issues is the recent address by T. R. Dawber entitled "Annual Discourse—Unproved Hypotheses" presented at the annual meeting of the Massachusetts Medical Society. Dawber did not consider exotic or esoteric topics. He simply asked for verification of the impressions widely held by physicians that (1) sodium intake is related to hypertension, (2) tonsillectomy prevents respiratory disease, (3) alcoholism is a disease and (4) fat intake is related to development of atherosclerosis.[5] If those four almost everyday opinions are not established, consider how many other elements of medical practice are in need of scientific study. As we consider the erection of an edifice for whole-person medicine, we must be careful not to build on a foundation of shifting sand—that is, on unverified hypotheses such as those in Dawber's list.

Is There a Secular Model for Whole-Person Medicine?

An additional feature of whole-person medicine should be of interest to those who plan medical curricula. It is the question, "Is there a nonsectarian whole-person medicine?" That is, is whole-person medicine necessarily Christian? If, as Robert Herrmann suggested, spiritual factors must be included with physical, environmental, cultural and emotional elements in the composite that is health, how can a curriculum sponsoring the whole-person concept be developed by the faculty of a secular medical school? It seems to me that this conference must face this issue head-on. It possibly represents one more example of the exclusiveness of the Christian position. Christians believe that we have a valid whole-person concept (whereas those who are not Christian believers cannot).

Herein may lie the greatest opportunity presented to Oral Roberts University, to Loma Linda University—and possibly to medical schools of Roman Catholic universities. Beginning from the Christian world-and-life view, a whole-person concept of health care can be appropriated, and a curriculum can be designed toward that end. Secular universities, by contrast, may find that difficult or even impossible. If so, all the leadership will have to come from the uniquely Christian schools. They can provide that leadership only in part through the training they offer their own students and house officers. Beside that they will have a responsibility to create models or standards of practice that can be adopted by Christian physicians who may have graduated from secular schools, but who recognize the advantages of the whole-person, explicitly Christian, philosophy of health care.

When I have my next bout of serious illness I hope to come under the care of a physician competent in whole-person medicine. But I hope equally fervently that he or she graduated from a school of medicine that has not forgotten how to train investigators and that is staffing its clinical departments with persons imaginative in research as well as in clinical care and teaching.

Notes

[1] Abraham Flexner, *Medical Education in the United States and Canada: A Report to the Carnegie Foundation for the Advancement of Teaching*, Bulletin No. 4 (New York, 1910).

[2] Abraham Flexner, *An Autobiography* (New York: Simon and Schuster, 1960).

[3] Flexner, *Medical Education*, p. 68.

[4] Roslyn S. Wolman, "A Tale of Two Colonial Cities: Inoculation against Smallpox in Philadelphia and in Boston," *Transactions and Studies of the Philadelphia College of Physicians*, 45 (1978), 338-47.

[5] T. R. Dawber, "Annual Discourse—Unproved Hypotheses," *New England Journal of Medicine*, 299 (1978), 452-58.

Chapter Five

To Heal and Be Healed: A Medical Student's Perspective

Robert M. Nelson

The health-care system in the United States is heading for an inevitable crisis. Many people, including physicians, are dissatisfied with the present system, which includes: increasing specialization and a resulting maldistribution of primary health care; advanced technology with the specter of "saving lives," while failing to "save people," and escalating costs; limited access and inadequate resources for underprivileged sectors of the population.[1] Medical technology has become an end in itself, with the focus on disease rather than on the patient.[2]

Often associated with such criticisms are varied views of the "true" aim of medicine, that is, the meaning of health. Popularly, to be healthy is to jog, to play tennis, to meditate and to be a vegetarian. During this time of flux in legislative health policy, our understanding of health and disease, and of the doctor's role in preventing disease and promoting health, may significantly affect the future of health care.

It is within this context and with a sense of hope toward the future that our discussion of whole-person medicine takes place. The discussion encompasses three areas corresponding to components of the relationship essential to clinical medicine: the physician-patient relationship. The three components are the physician, the patient and the surrounding context or health-care system. For example, from a patient's perspective, concerns center on the needs arising from a person's psychological and social system when under the impact of disease. Patients evaluate the health-care delivery system on the basis of whether or not those needs are being recognized and provided for.

One can recite a litany of deficiencies as well as accomplishments for our present system. In addressing the deficiencies, however, the physician is seen as a component of the delivery system and not as a separate individual within the therapeutic relationship. The physician's training is thus examined as to its adequacy in areas such as nutrition and geriatrics; the physician is blamed for faults of the system that arise, for example, from the "fee for service" mentality.

This essay will consider two issues: first, the concept of health that lies behind all discussions of whole-person medicine; and second, the physician, not simply as an aspect of the health-care delivery system, but as a whole person striving to heal others.

What is Health?
Individuals who support the concept of whole-person medicine as being useful for the orientation of our health-care system seem to be tacitly agreeing with the definition of health given by the World Health Organization (WHO): "Health is a state of complete physical, mental and social well-being and not merely the absence of disease or infirmity."[3] Adopted by the 1946 International Health Conference as part of the preamble to the constitution of the WHO, that all-inclusive statement has often been criticized yet seems to endure. A brief survey of the criticisms is useful[4] as we formulate our Christian view of health, that is, of whole-person medicine.

Is the definition of health too vague to be useful? A broad criticism, usually from so-called pragmatists, is that the concept *health* is too vague for its definition to be of any practical value for the medical profession. Even the most pragmatic judgment, however, presupposes certain values and orientations. Often behind such a critique is a belief that physicians should limit their goal to the treatment of disease, that is, to the removal of negative constraints, rather than fostering a positive ideal of health. Limiting the physician's role to treating disease gives rise to two problems.

First, though we believe that by our modern biomedical determinants we have limited disease to the realm of "hard fact," that has not been[5] and is not now always true.[6] The concept of disease can easily transgress the boundaries of descriptive scientific evaluation to that of prescriptive moral valuation, as amply demonstrated by the misuse of psychiatric diagnosis in the Soviet Union.[7] Similar problems arise when medical parameters of disease are applied to an ostensibly healthy population, as in screening programs. Not only are there "normal" people who fall outside two standard deviations from the mean, but there are clearly "sick" people who feel that they are perfectly healthy. Who is correct?[8] Where is the line, if there is one, between objective and subjective criteria of disease?

Second, to limit the physician's role to the treatment of disease maintains the status quo and thus perpetuates the present system with its various problems—since the treatment of disease is indeed the system's forte. Yet people want to be healthy, not merely free from disease, and rightly or wrongly they come to physicians to find health. This societal desire for health compels the medical profession to re-examine and possibly abandon its conceptual limitation of health care to the removal of disease. Simply stated, our society wants physicians to provide health care, not just disease treatment. To ignore such expectations is to deny our professional responsibility.

Other criticisms of the WHO definition. Many people recognize that a widely used definition of a term as crucial as *health* can have important implications. Daniel Callahan cites four basic objections.

First, by equating social problems with health problems, the definition renders all human well-being a medical problem, suitable to medical intervention. At the least, the WHO statement emphasizes the common-sense observation that social well-being is not merely the absence of disease or infirmity. One could reverse the logic of that equation, however, and see the WHO definition of health as defining all medical diseases as social ills, and not vice versa. Medical problems are thus rendered suitable to social intervention; such intervention is commonly accepted in child abuse, infant "failure-to-thrive," alcoholism and occupational diseases. In that sense, the definition of health is rather trivial; it simply reminds one of the multifarious etiologies and far-reaching implications of a disease beyond the mere physical health of one individual. Yet, as Callahan points out, the WHO intends more than that: it wants health to be a fundamental precondition for peace. It could be argued that without health there will not be peace; yet recent times have certainly shown that health does not bring peace.

The problem of human happiness is often not health but human finitude, that is, the inevitable limitations of reality in spite of infinite human desires and aspirations. In seeking to broaden our concept of health, we must retain the important distinction between health care as meeting deeply felt human needs and health care as a utopian panacea.

Second, Callahan points out, the concept of health in the WHO definition, blurs lines of responsibility. It gives the medical profession the task of providing for "social well-being" by treating "social disease." An example is the widespread incarceration of criminals in mental institutions rather than in prisons.

Third, Callahan continues, the other side of the issue of medical responsibility is loss of patient responsibility. One aspect of the traditional sick role is the nonresponsibility or blamelessness ascribed to those who are ill. If all mental, physical and social disorders become defined as "sickness," it becomes difficult if not impossible to ascribe any freedom or responsibility to ailing individuals.

Responsibility and power are two issues that need to be investigated further. Ascription of nonresponsibility to the sick person was most appropriate in the era of infectious diseases where an individual was struck down suddenly and was often unable to take preventive measures. Yet new knowledge of the pathogenesis of disease, the prevention of infectious and nutritional disease, and the prevalence of so-called diseases of lifestyle lead us to ask if the concept of the patient's non-responsibility for disease retains its purpose and applicability. Related to that issue is the interplay between the concepts of disease and unhealth. It is often said that the opposite of health is not disease, but unhealth. If that is so, can we ascribe responsibility to people for their unhealth, but not for their disease? It strikes me that such a distinction would be impossible to maintain in practice.

Related to a conceptual shift from disease to unhealth is a related shift in the locus of power. When the patient was not responsible, the physician was. If the patient is now responsible, where does that leave the physician? As the focus of our health-care delivery shifts from the treatment of disease to the nurturing of health, a shift of power from the physician as provider, to the patient and society as consumer, is inevitable. Not all the power will shift; the relationship will remain complex. Yet, practically speaking, there will be a shift in the allocation of funds for health care away from the delivery of disease-treatment and toward programs targeted for the provision of health.

Given such shifts in responsibility and power, criticisms of an inclusive definition of health as "blurring lines of responsibility" can adequately be countered. The resistance toward the concept of whole-person medicine shown by some of those presently holding power and responsibility also becomes understandable.

Fourth, Callahan concludes, critics such as Thomas Szasz have recognized that moving the concept of health from the medical to the moral arena entails certain dangers. What could not be done in the name of morality can now be done in the name of health: "Human beings labelled, incarcerated, and dismissed for their failure to toe the line of 'normalcy' and 'sanity.' "[9] As all human disorders become defined as forms of illness, health becomes normative—something everyone ought to have in order to live at peace with themselves and others.

Extension of the concept of health from physical well-being

to include mental and social well-being rests on various psychological, sociopolitical and moral assumptions that are not universally accepted in our pluralistic society. Though we may all agree that health means physical, mental, social and spiritual well-being, we will often disagree on what constitutes well-being. Such disagreements can be so fundamental that our concepts of health are incompatible, although each could in all good conscience agree with the WHO definition. Opposed to such conceptual confusion, Callahan chooses to limit the meaning of health to "physical well-being" in an attempt to make the concept useful by eliminating controversial assumptions.

Yet limiting the concept of health is not the only approach to the problem of the implicit moral judgments behind such a concept. Another solution would be to allow extension of the concept of health but recognize as essential to the concept the self-referential nature of the necessary moral judgments as well as the above-mentioned shifts in responsibility and power. As Arthur Dyck has pointed out in chapter 2, the physician-patient relationship is founded on a covenant of mutual trust, a trust predicated on respect for other persons as equals. Included are respect for their moral judgments and, in particular, respect for their judgment about what constitutes their physical, mental, social and spiritual well-being.

It is one thing to allow individuals to identify their needs; it is another to take a notion of well-being and screen a population for those who are "ill." To prevent such abuse, the notion of health and well-being must be strictly self-referential out of a respect for the moral autonomy of individuals. It may be that as a society we will make the hard decision that certain "needs" identified by people cannot be met. Yet such decisions should not be justified by excluding those needs from a definition of health that would then function normatively.

Though Callahan's solution removes ambiguities, is it adequate to meet the impending crisis in health care? No. The crisis arises not out of a misunderstanding of the term, but from a recognition that the present disease-oriented system falls short of meeting basic human health needs. Can we truly say that our health-care system is adequate when the leading cause of death among black teen-agers in the United States is violence? Not without making a mockery of the word *adequate*. As hopelessly abstract as the WHO definition of health may be, its longevity is perhaps due to the recognition that our health, or perhaps our wholeness, encompasses all of the interrelated aspects of our being: physical, mental, social and spiritual. Rather than running from problems that such an all-inclusive concept presents, we should face them, refusing to capitulate to the reductionist tendencies of modern medicine and society. Though Callahan's criticisms are well taken, they can be responded to without abandoning a wholistic approach to health care.

The physician as a whole person. The concept of whole-person medicine includes more than an analysis of the patient as person and the subsequent needs to be met by the health-care system and thus by the physician. It should include the physician not simply as the provider of care but also as one cared for. To see the physician only as a provider is to see him or her as simply an aspect of the system and not as a whole person working within the system. If being fully human requires caring for and being cared for, these two aspects of whole personhood need to be considered for both patient and physician. The above-mentioned emphasis on patients' moral autonomy permits them to care for themselves, rather than simply being cared for. Now we must turn to consider the physician as being cared for, rather than simply providing care. Though I am limiting my discussion here to physicians, the same considerations are important for any provider within the present health-care delivery system.

Concern for the physician as a whole person rests on two main considerations. First, the issue arises of whether a physician is able to meet the needs of patients if his or her needs are not being provided for. Will physicians, for example, be sensitive to the emotional overlay of disease and its impact on a patient's life if during their medical training they have consistently denied or suppressed the emotional impact of disease in order to function within a system that rewards technical competence at the expense of personal development?

Second, concern for the physician as a whole person entails more than just his or her ability to provide for patients. It must also include concern for the physician as a person outside the system in which he or she works. This second aspect acknowledges that as the health-care consumer cries out to be recognized as a person and not simply as a patient, so the physician desires to be seen as a person within the role of health-care provider. That desire, if actualized, would place certain demands on the system within which the physician works and trains, as well as on the expectations and attitudes of people looking to the medical profession for care.

Why are the rates of alcoholism, drug abuse, suicide and divorce among physicians higher than among almost any other professional group? Is that a situation which must necessarily exist?

The physical and psychological stresses of medical training and practice are well known, yet the tragedy is how easily such pressures are accepted as being necessary to the training of a physician—as if medical school and residency were rites of passage or purification before one can enter the "holy of holies." Certainly some of the pressures are the inevitable result of long hours and large amounts of material to be learned, plus the strain of dealing, day in and day out, with sick and dying people. But the pressures can be decreased by (1) providing ways for medical students, residents and attending physicians to deal with their emotions and stress, and (2) avoiding certain counter-productive attitudes.

My experience as a hospital chaplain, for example, convinced me of the need for broad-based pastoral and psychological care for physicians, nurses and hospital staff.[10] Informal group sessions as well as individual counseling should be available throughout medical school and residency training. In addition, proper grievance procedures should be set up so that educational abuses can be identified and corrected. Regrettably, the attitude exists among some resident and attending physicians that since they were mistreated during their education, they will mistreat others. Often that attitude is exacerbated by a misplaced competitive instinct. The first step toward humanizing medicine will be for physicians to treat one another as persons and for medical students to learn that they are respected as unique individuals.

The humanizing of medicine, however, will require more than a simple change of attitude. We must take a hard look at our health-care institutions and the stresses placed on those working within them. Is it appropriate to expect third-year medical students to be on call every third night? Certainly they will need to be on call at some point in the future, but is it really necessary during their first clinical exposure? Or, if they have been on all night, should they be able to take the next morning or afternoon off? Most medical schools now have their fourth-year students do clinical rotations as "sub-interns" to prepare for their first year of residency. That policy would seem to obviate a need for excessive night call during the third year.

Another important issue is the effect of medical training and practice on social and family life. Two fundamental human endeavors are work and family, yet we have driven a wedge between them by the demands our modern medical institutions place on us. Can the isolation that results be considered at all "healthy"?

Answers to such problems will come about only through grappling with the issues, guided by the conviction that the whole person of the physician should be considered in the structuring of our health-care institutions.

It distresses me that so often only the physician-as-provider is considered (that is, the physician as healer) and not the physician as needing to be healed. As a human person, I may be in as much need of healing as the human person to whom I, as physician, would minister.

In conclusion, the basic insight of the WHO definition of health as encompassing all aspects of our well-being ought to guide the education and practice of physicians as well as the structuring of health-care institutions. Essential to that guiding function is the principle of the self-referential nature of moral judgments concerning health or well-being, so that health and the health-care system will not become an insidious form of institutional control over individual behavior. Concern for the patient's moral autonomy is grounded in respect for his or her personhood. A similar respect must be shown for the person of the physician and other health-care providers. Thus we must recognize our fundamental equality and mutuality as individual persons within a context intended to promote healing and come to appreciate the need for healing and the gift of healing on the part of all concerned.

Finally, as Christians (both as physicians and patients), we are called to a healing ministry of the whole person as both body and spirit—a ministry best exemplified by the Lord Jesus in his life and death. During his lifetime Jesus often concerned himself with physical healing as a sign of the breaking in of the kingdom of God and also as a counterpart to spiritual healing through faith. His atoning death combines spiritual restoration with the dimension of physical healing. We see this graphically in Matthew 8:17 where Jesus' healing of Peter's mother-in-law is closely tied to the messianic image of Jesus as the suffering servant of Isaiah 53. Consistent with the Lord's ministry, physical healing played an important role in the ministry of the early church (see Mk. 16:14-18).

I suspect that everyone has an intuitive sense of the meaning of health as encompassing their physical well-being (by the most up-to-date medical standards), their sense of community and the values they hold dear. With our values and communities disintegrating, we need a better understanding not of the meaning of health but rather of what it means to be a healer and to be healed. As Christian physicians, we need to care for and to serve our patients and to love them in the fullest sense of the meaning of *agape*—those are the root concepts behind our word *therapeutics*. To be sensitive to the wounds of both a bruised body and a bruised spirit, and through God's Spirit to heal and be healed—that is the true meaning of health.

Health is a process, not a state. It is a mutual enterprise, the movement of God's Spirit within our human community.

Notes

[1] John H. Knowles, M.D., ed., "Doing Better and Feeling Worse: Health in the United States," *Daedalus,* 106 (Winter 1977).

[2] Leon R. Kass, "Regarding the End of Medicine and the Pursuit of Health," *The Public Interest,* No. 40 (Summer 1975).

[3] *Official Record World Health Organization,* 2, p. 100.

[4] Daniel Callahan, "The WHO Definition of Health," *The Hastings Center Studies,* 1, No. 3 (1973).

[5] H. Tristram Engelhardt, Jr., "The Disease of Masturbation: Values and the Concept of Disease," *Bulletin of the History of Medicine,* 48, No. 2 (Summer 1974).

[6] Christopher Boorse, "On the Distinction between Disease and Illness," *Philosophy and Public Affairs,* 5, No. 1 (1975).

[7] Sidney Bloch, "Psychiatry as Ideology in the USSR," *Journal of Medical Ethics,* 4, No. 3 (September 1978).

[8] Stephen R. Kellert, "A Sociocultural Concept of Health and Illness," *The Journal of Medicine and Philosophy,* 1, No. 3 (1976).

[9] Callahan.

[10] David C. Duncombe, Arthur M. Gershkoff and Robert M. Nelson, "Medical Students in CPE," *The Journal of Pastoral Care,* 32, No. 3 (September 1978).

Chapter Six

Educating the Christian Physician

E. D. Pellegrino

To be a physician is to be committed to a noble ideal. To be a Christian physician is to add dimensions of inspiration and aspiration that elevate the ideal immeasurably. The Christian physician is called to imitate an ineffable model, an incarnate God whose own ministry was inseparable from healing.[1]

Yet no vocation, even healing, is uniquely Christian. Nor does being a Christian alone suffice. Only in the creative fusion of two existential states, being a Christian and being a physician, is it possible to realize that ideal. That fusion, and the special obligations it entails, are the unique call to which Christians who are teaching, studying and practicing medicine must individually and collectively respond.

Today this challenge is extraordinarily difficult. We are still seeking how best to teach and practice medical humanism of the secular kind.[2] Can we even hope then to teach what it means to witness authentically to Christ through the profession of medicine? Even in those few schools under religious auspices there are no formal models for educating Christian physicians. What teaching occurs is largely by example. Christians themselves have allowed the act of healing to become progressively secularized. They and their patients readily accommodate a widening separation of healing from faith and ministry. Some even seem apologetic and reticent about being Christian physicians, thus isolating faith from life.

These responses are the predictable result of misunderstanding the strength and the limitations of the conception of modern medicine as science. The undeniably dramatic and indispensable contributions of scientific methodology to therapeutics foster an understandable hubris. Specific cure for every known illness is the ambitious aim of medical science. The temptation to believe that medicine can stand alone is very strong. What, we are asked, can religion add to such wondrous achievements?

Some fear that zealous adherence to Christian values might lead to neglect of science, to passivity in the face of illness and death and to inhibition of the free pursuit of knowledge. There are also dangers, it is thought, of using the vulnerable state of the sick person to proselytize. Finally, religion undeniably introduces complex moral questions which do impede the "free" use of medical science to determine the future of humanity.

Although medicine in America and in the West has long had strong religious roots, medical ethics are being secularized. In a morally pluralistic society it is difficult to agree on the resolution of specific medical moral dilemmas. Competence and legalism rather than ideals of obligation and service have come to dominate professional codes, as the recently proposed revisions of the code of the AMA attest.[3]

We urgently need a reconstruction of our codes of medical morality. Such a reconstruction is not likely, ever again, to be religiously inspired. At best we can hope for a common substratum of obligations justified philosophically in the nature of the physician-patient relationship.[4] The Christian physician will have to build on that substratum those higher levels of inspiration and obligation called for by the revelation of the Christian message.

I cite this litany of obstacles because even Christian physicians use them as justification for not addressing the issue of how to educate the Christian physician. Yet the Christian medical teacher who ignores that challenge risks serious hypocrisy and can frustrate the fullness of the Christian experience in students. The teacher thereby derogates the enormous power of Christian humanism to reverse the alarming trend of contemporary medicine to become alienated from the humane purposes to which it is ordained. Finally, he or she deprives patients of the healing powers of faith, powers every true Christian must draw upon.

How is the Christian physician to be educated? What is to be taught and how? What is feasible in a secular institution? What more is possible and demanded in a school specifically dedicated to the education of Christian physicians?

I shall address these questions in three stages: first, by examining what it means to be a physician in purely human terms—the terms of secular humanism; then by seeing what must be added to the human ideal by being a Christian— the terms of Christian humanism; and, finally, having defined the educational goal, by seeing how it is to be pursued.

Before examining these three issues, I feel impelled to acknowledge the dedication to high ideals of morality and practice by those Jewish, Muslim and nonbelieving men and women who follow their own perception of the good physician. They too care deeply for their patients as suffering fellow humans. Often enough, they share with Christians a loving concern for those they attend. As a Christian I would surely be out of order trying to define what additional dimensions the religious beliefs of non-Christians bring to being a physician. It is what Christianity specifically brings that must be my concern.

The Physician as Physician—Reason Unaided by Faith

In a series of papers I have tried to define what it means to be a physician on the basis of a philosophical inquiry into the nature of medicine and the physician-patient relationship.[5] I can only summarize my position here.

The act specific to medicine, that which makes it medicine and thereby distinguishes it from both science and art, is a decision about what is right and good for a particular patient. The central and irreducible concern of medicine is *this* patient, *now*, with *this* set of needs, arising out of *this* particular illness. Science is necessary to specify the causes of the patient's illness, to determine what modes of therapy are available, which ones are effective and how safe they are. Art is required to assure perfection in carrying out the decision of a skillful examination, operation or manipulation. But the essence of medicine is neither art nor science. It is the practical decision, taken in the best interest of a particular person, not in the interest of new knowledge, of society, or of the physician.

Once we speak of a *right* and *good* action we are squarely in the realm of morals, the realm of what *ought* to be done. Medicine, therefore, is at its center a moral enterprise. I have construed it in the Aristotelian sense as a practical virtue, a *Recta ratio agibilium.*[6] The physician's obligations arise out of two factors: (1) In undertaking to treat a patient he or she promises to act in that patient's interest, that is, to take the right and good healing action: (2) The physician makes that promise within a special human relationship, confronting another human being in a state of special vulnerability, the state of illness.

Persons who are ill are human beings in a state of compromised or wounded humanity. They have lost to varying degrees the distinctly human possibilities of free and rational decision making about themselves and their bodies. Persons who are ill do not know what is wrong. They do not have the skill to heal themselves. They can decide what is "best" only on the advice of another human being. The physician's act of "profession" implies that he or she will do everything in the patient's best interest. That act promises that the wounded humanity of ill persons will be healed—that information sufficient to make an informed choice will be provided, that the procedures will be competently and safely performed, that the patient's values, his or her assessment of what is worthwhile, rather than the physician's, will be respected.

In purely human terms, leaving religious imperatives aside for the moment, just being a physician imposes obligations of a special character. The special vulnerability of the experience of being ill demands that the physician's obligations transcend self-interest to a degree not demanded of other professions. That is why moral dimensions were recognized so early in the history of medicine.

At first, medical morality was simply like that of a good craftsman—a competent job must be done. In addition, a kind and sympathetic demeanor was required to assure cooperation and establish a good reputation. Those were the elements of the early Greek notion of *philanthropia*—not charity or love in the Christian sense.[7] The nobler sentiments often attributed to Greek medicine were later infusions from Stoicism and the precepts of Christian, Jewish and Muslim religions. Each modified and then adopted the Hippocratic ethic and thus universalized it for physicians in the West.

The middle and late Stoics raised medical morality to noble heights. Scribonius Largus, physician to the Emperor Claudius and a follower of the moral philosophy of Panaetius and Cicero, first introduced the word *profession* in relation to medicine. Scribonius was also the first to suggest that the morality of the physician was specifically related to the nature of the profession of medicine. He went so far as to use the words *humanitas* (love of humanity) and *misericordia* (mercy). These, he argued, were obligations intrinsic to being a physician. Without them the practitioner could not be a member of the profession but rather became a traitor or deserter.[8]

Some of the later Stoics, like Sarapion and Libanius (the latter in his address to the young physician), went even further. They specifically admonished the physician to treat the patient as a brother. Thus the Stoics saw medicine as a vocation, as Christians do. But they derived the obligations of that vocation from the nature of a calling voluntarily assumed. The nobility of the Stoic sentiments is remarkable. They represent the highest expression of what it is to be a physician to which natural reason, unenlightened by revelation, can attain. Admittedly, these pagan writers lived in the early years of the Christian era, and it is conceivable that they imbibed some of the teachings of the Christian community. Their historical and textual connections with Christianity are presently not established. Whatever their source, the lofty ideals of medical morality propounded by the Stoics were a distinct advance over Hippocratic ethics. Such ideals remain a model of medical humanism still uniting all, religious and nonreligious, who profess to be humanistic healers.

The Religious and the Christian Physician
With such high ideals, what more can be added by a religious dimension? Since even the word *love* was used by the later Stoics, is anything more needed? What additional dimensions of obligation does any religion add to those required by the act of profession and by the nature of the physician-patient relationship?

First, I must say what I mean by *religion*. I refer to any system of belief that derives its justification from some principle, power or force outside human beings, which requires of them certain duties not self-generated and which may or may not also require certain ritual practices. The difference between religion and nonreligion is an act of faith, or nonfaith, in a power beyond humanity. This definition is intentionally broad enough to encompass all varieties of belief. It underscores the distinction between what is required of the physician as physician by secular humanism and what is added by any belief.

The religious believer who unites belief with profession incurs all the responsibilities contained in Scribonius's Stoic ideal. But he or she must also be faithful to an additional set of values, inspirations and practices attributable to the transcendental principle believed in. The shape and meaning of the Stoic ideals of *humanitas* and *misericordia* are therefore specifically modulated by the world view each religion imposes.

For the religious believer, all morality receives its ultimate justification from a source outside and superior to humankind. The religious person cannot hold that morality is self-justifying. Certain obligations are deducible by reason alone, it is true, but the highest display of human moral agency demands adjustments to the higher principle in which the religious person has faith.

For the Christian, that higher dimension is revealed in the gospel of Jesus Christ, whose irruption into human history redeemed humanity, fulfilled the prophecies of the Old Testament and forever altered the meaning of human relationships. All who follow Christ must love God as Father; all human beings are potential brothers and sisters. Every incident in the life of Jesus exemplified Christian love and charity. The Beatitudes teach explicitly how being a Christian differs from even the highest expressions of morality in the Old Testament or in the best pagan philosophers.

Søren Kierkegaard's question, "Who is a Christian?" must be answered daily by every Christian and every church. The Christian is committed to the special way of love and charity exemplified by Christ. That way must illuminate the Christian's every action and thought. He or she must become a partner in Christ's ministry to the world. With the church, the Christian is called to evangelize, witness, teach and announce the good news.

Christian physicians have in Christ a more explicit model to inspire them than any other profession except the clergy. Healing was Jesus' daily task. He healed body and soul; in him healing and salvation were one. Healing exemplified his love for men and women in the most concrete way. The Greek word *sōzein* meant both to heal and to save. Christ had compassion on the vulnerability of the sick. He knew the meaning of bodily suffering, and himself tasted it to the fullest in the garden of Gethsemane and on the cross.

If they are to follow Christ, healing for Christian physicians cannot ever be anything other than ministry. It cannot ever be merely science or even public service. Physicians heal insofar as medical knowledge allows. But they must also care for and feel for the sick, whether medical means are adequate or not. Christian compassion means to "suffer with" those who suffer.

The Christian ministry of healing is not reserved for those

who can pay, or for the educated, the grateful, the clean, for "our kind of people," or for those who "help themselves." It must be extended to all who suffer; it must be given with love to all, or it is not Christian. Christian physicians are authentic only if they unite their Christianity inseparably with their healing.

That inseparability must be manifest alongside scientific competence, which complements and supplements it. The two need never be in conflict. Yet Christian physicians should acknowledge their own dependence on God and recognize him as the ultimate source of all the wonders science uncovers for human benefit. Christian physicians are not afraid to pray with and for their patients, to acknowledge God's participation in all their healing acts, to look to him when human measures fail, and always to help a patient find him. Praying with patients and their families is not to deny science or even to weaken our zeal for its fullest application. It is to recognize human limitations, to ask God's blessing on the physician's action and to place the patient, the physician and medicine in proper relationship to God. To minimize the physician's hubris is not to derogate science but simply to place it in the order of God's creation as a great good but not as a universal ideology that supplants religion and faith.

How many of us who claim to be Christian physicians, and how many institutions that claim to be Christian, could stand the scrutiny of Jesus? How would he respond to seeing us on our ward rounds, in the office, at the board meeting, in the business office or the emergency room? The nobility of the ideal of being a Christian physician or a Christian hospital is what makes its fulfillment so exquisitely difficult and its failure so scandalous.

Who would not wither before the gaze of Christ were he to see our fee setting, our bill collecting, our self-justifying unavailability, our putdown of the ignorant, our transgression of the values of our patients, our standardizing, mathematicizing, pragmatic assembly-line clinics? We have only to think of his anger with the moneychangers in the temple to remember that hypocrisy was his special enemy.

Christian physicians cannot ever be satisfied with mere adherence to a professional code. They seek perfection in Christ. Whereas reason may argue for or against abortion, euthanasia, or test-tube babies, Christians must resolve such dilemmas in the light of what Christian belief teaches. Christians have to reflect constantly on their ministry of healing, not simply as an obligation arising from the nature of a human relationship—as a philosopher would argue the case—but as an obligation of a believer in the redemptive message of Jesus Christ.

For the denominational Christian, and I will say a word only about the Roman Catholic denomination, there is the additional dimension of the particular construal the church places on the message of Christ. The Roman Catholic is a member of a community, the mystical body uniting all its members in a community of ministry which vitalizes their individual ministries. That community is a source not only of special grace but also of special obligation.

The denominational Christian then works, thinks, acts within a multileveled matrix—he or she has obligations simply as a physician, then as a physician committed to a religious principle of justification beyond the human, then as a Christian and, finally, as a Christian of a particular persuasion.

Conferences like this one help us to explore these several levels of moral agency together, and thus to understand the differing obligations each of us assumes in our healing ministry. Christian health workers sorely need a common code of Christian medical morality equal to the complex challenges posed by our secular and morally pluralistic society. Such a moral code would first set out the obligations all Christian physicians share simply by being followers of Christ. Each denomination could add to that base in modular fashion its specific obligations with respect to the common moral dilemmas in which there may be disagreement. To elaborate such a common code we must first separate and identify our philosophic and theological formulations of medical morality as this essay suggests.

I do not believe that a professional code justified only

philosophically will ever assure those who are ill the dedicated service the physician owes them. Every trend of modern medicine—its exploitation of technology, its institutionalization, its bureaucratization, its cost, its power to alter man biologically and behaviorally—ultimately accentuates the need for a religious source of morality. A totally adequate medical morality is not derivable from general morality nor is morality itself fully justifiable on philosophical considerations alone.

What Can Be Taught and How?

I have tried to locate the Christian physician in relationship to medical morality because I cannot speak about teaching until I am clear about what is to be taught. What I have tried to show thus far is that we are required to prepare a physician who is both scientifically competent and an authentic Christian healer. We must prepare the student for a Christian ministry grounded simultaneously in professional competence and the manifestation and proclamation of the Christian faith. The medical school that sets such a goal for itself must undertake the spiritual formation of its medical students as vigorously as it does the preparation of its ordained ministers. Professional capability must be interwoven with Christian witness to form a unity.

The problem is compounded enormously by the fact that the medical schools of the world are overwhelmingly secular and usually openly antipathetic to any notion of religious formation, often on constitutional grounds. Even those medical schools under the aegis of Christian universities have thus far only indirectly addressed the problem of Christian formation as an institutional policy.

My recommendations are therefore divided into two parts: what can be done in schools under Christian auspices, and what can be done in secular institutions. I wish to underscore that I am definitely not being critical of schools that have not done what I shall outline. I have been asked to say what can be done, and so I will focus on the minimal requirements which would have to be met to enable each student to learn what it is to be a Christian physician.

In Christian medical schools. Let us turn first to a medical school under Christian auspices which consciously establishes the teaching of Christian physicians as an institutional objective. What are minimal requirements to attaining that end?

The first, the indispensable and the most difficult requirement is to provide teaching by example and behavior. What could be simpler or more difficult for individual faculty members of the institution? What is demanded is that we be Christian ourselves, that we live the ministry of healing every moment of every day. That entails, at least, exhibiting those levels of obligation I have just outlined as a requisite for the fusion of Christianity with medicine. Surely, if the student is to be convinced of the probity of the Christian ministry of healing, he or she will expect that the search for God and Christ will be taken seriously, that faith is sustained and deepened, that a concern for justice and mercy is manifest and that a dedication to religious and moral values enters into each clinical decision.

To be authentic as Christian physicians, teachers must demonstrate that we care for the patient, that we place the patient's needs above our own convenience and comfort, that we wear our authority and knowledge humbly, that we teach, explain and be patient and sensitive to every nuance of behavior which might introduce even a trace of humiliation for the vulnerable person who is ill. To turn one's back thoughtlessly to a patient even in a single instance undoes hours of lectures about Christian charity and lets in the odor of hypocrisy which students can detect in even infinitesimal amounts.

The Christian physician must evidence a sense of the inequality of the relationship between one who has knowledge and another who needs that knowledge to be healed. The Christian physician feels the vulnerability, the wounded humanity, the humiliation, the nakedness of body and soul that illness brings. The Christian feels these things along with the person who is ill. That is what compassion means. The Christian makes every decision, performs every medical act with this existential meaning of illness always in mind.

Ministry is service infused by the invigorating powers of faith, hope and love. How authentic is that mission if our competence is suspect? How authentic, when we hurry the patient, chide, scold or ridicule? How authentic when we rush off to our amusement or recreation, or make ourselves "unavailable" at this or that time? How authentic when we justify our fees and our procedures by our selfish desires for a certain style of life or even by the ingeniously inane claim that every other physician does that too?

Those who hope to teach what it is to be a Christian physician must themselves exemplify an impossibly difficult idea. They cannot be defeated by the perfection of the model they are called on to imitate, the healing ministry of Christ himself. The teacher is destined forever to fall short of the model. Yet even in falling short we can make our lesson clear if we pursue the goal with conscious purpose, humility and clear intent.

Because of these difficulties, teaching by example must be supplemented by formal instruction in certain cognitive essentials. The student must comprehend the intellectual foundations of Christian practice and morals, especially as they pertain to clinical decision making. Formal teaching in ethics, theology and philosophy is crucial if the Christian physician is to understand and justify clinical decisions, especially the value questions those decisions so often encompass.

I argued above that the medical act is a moral one, that it involves a choice of what ought to be done for a particular patient and that it must be taken in the patient's interest. Christian physicians must, therefore, take account of the values and the conscience of the patient, even when those values are opposed to their own. They must respect the patient's exercise of moral agency. They cannot manipulate, force or ignore the patient's personal moral choices without becoming less Christian. This limitation demands a careful understanding by Christians of their own value system, and of where it conflicts on essential points with the patient's. Christians are required to know when they must kindly, respectfully and firmly dissociate themselves from a particular patient whose definitions of what is right and good violate Christian morality.

Important decisions of this kind cannot safely rest on feelings or on someone else's example alone. Each physician must understand his or her own conscience, what moral principles are in conflict and where compromise can be made and where it cannot. The systematic study of philosophy, theology and ethics enables the student to locate himself or herself as Christian with reference to the increasingly frequent moral dilemmas and conflicts of obligations which we face today. Faith and a reasonable understanding of that faith are the necessary accoutrements of the educated Christian.

The teaching of ethics, philosophy and theology cannot be left to medical teachers alone, no matter how enlightened or well-intentioned. Those courses must be taught as rigorously as the scientific foundations of medicine. They are best taught by professional theologians and philosophers in the clinical setting, by the case method, and related to the concrete dilemmas of medical decision making. My decade of experience in teaching the humanities in American medical schools has convinced me that cooperative teaching by clinicians and humanists is the most effective method.[9]

Christian physicians need to understand their beliefs as educated persons. They treat people of all beliefs and persuasions. They are called to be witnesses to all of them, intellectually as well as in their behavior. Theology cannot safely be isolated from medicine. Cardinal Newman once pointed out: "religious truth is not only a portion but a condition of general knowledge. To blot it out is nothing short, if I may so speak, of unravelling the web of university education."[10]

The complementarity of faith and reason does not require that science become subservient to theology or that faith replace competence. Every class in anatomy need not be interspersed with readings from the Scriptures (as some seem to suppose). That kind of *reductio ad absurdum* is the easy refuge of the secularist who cannot comprehend that both faith and competence are demanded of Christian physicians.

The formal teaching of theology and ethics does not mean

that physicians become amateur theologians or replace the minister. Nor does it require that they use their theology as an instrument of apologetics or for proselytizing. To take such advantage of the vulnerability of the sick, even for so good a purpose, is to violate Christian charity and the patient-physician covenant.

Still, Christian physicians are bound to attend to body, mind and spirit. They must recognize needs in all three realms. A theology of illness strengthens both physician and patient to confront illness as an opportunity for spiritual growth. Such a theology is a source of meaning and explanation not available to the secular humanist. Without usurping the functions of a minister, students should be taught to encourage and facilitate them. They must learn to avoid the temptation to extend their technical and legal authority beyond the bedside to moral and religious questions.

Students must also be taught to be Christian in their mode of evangelization as in the message they bring to the sick and dying. The lines separating facilitation and coercion, persuasion and manipulation are too fine for advance determination. Christian physicians must recognize that healing, bodily and spiritual, are never unilateral. Healing is grounded in the human relationship binding one in need and one who professes to help. Freedom of each person is crucial to authentic healing.

If students are to be taught optimally, the formal and informal teaching I have described must be reinforced daily by the institutions within which they are taught. The medical school and the hospital must exhibit a corporate and collective concern for the Christian healing ministry in every one of its operations. Its behavior, like that of the individual teacher, must be Christian. All patients are entitled to charity, mercy and justice. To be a Christian institution demands the same behavior of the collectivity that I described earlier for the individual.

Being a Christian institution is far more difficult than being a Christian individual. It is much easier to shift responsibility, to do a "Pontius Pilate" act. Who, for example, decides—and how—to resolve the conflicts between fiscal soundness and a patient's needs? Do we treat each other, our workers and our patients with Christian love and charity? Does the institution concern itself with social justice in health care? Is such care truly available and accessible to all in need? Stringent obligations are assumed by any hospital that declares itself to be a Christian institution. Elsewhere I have outlined some of the obligations of a Catholic hospital.[11]

The same obligation to practice Christian morality binds a Christian medical school. Certain ethical obligations bind all medical schools by virtue of their special function in society.[12] Additional obligations are imposed on any medical school under religious or Christian auspices. Such a school is required to be Christian in its treatment of its major constituencies, patients, students and faculty. At a minimum that means teaching students their moral obligations to patients and to society, providing opportunity for their personal spiritual growth, placing the needs of patients above the needs of teaching and research whenever they are in conflict, and responding to the needs of the poor, the afflicted and the disadvantaged who are under the care of the faculty and students.

Much of the dehumanization medical students feel and see in the process of education and house-staff training would be ameliorated if medical schools were truly Christian in their institutional morality.

Yet serious difficulties arise in establishing any uniform set of principles to share collective behavior. In our society the principles of academic freedom, civil rights and participatory democracy are important. How does any institution, medical school or hospital assure that it is Christian? Does it limit its faculty and staff to Christians? How does it deal with the difference in value systems of those it treats and of those who serve it? Issues of constitutionality, inappropriate for discussion here, would be relevant to any attempt to develop an authentic sense of institutional Christian commitment.

Such difficulties notwithstanding, one principle is irreducible: to teach an ideal as lofty as that of the Christian physician, we must teach and practice everything in the spirit of Christ's own healing ministry. We must follow the motto of Pope Pius X, *"Instaurare Omnia in Christo."* No school or hospital will attain perfection in the practice of that ideal. We are redeemed, but we will never be perfect in this world. We have an incomparable model to guide us. The model of Christ the Healer transcends even the loftiest sentiments of naturalistically derived medical moralities.

The challenge to medical schools and hospitals professedly Christian is being met in many ways by schools under religious auspices. My message to them is that they must reflect continually, critically and analytically on whether or not they are as close to the ideal as they can be. They should ask themselves what Christ might say if he witnessed their daily work.

In secular medical schools.   In a secular medical school, of course, we cannot demand institutional commitment of the kind I have outlined. We can demand only what is philosophically justifiable through human reason unilluminated by revelation. Certain obligations, derivable from the nature of medicine and of the physician-patient relationship, apply to any institution of healing or teaching. Even here, though, we need a new, philosophically justifiable, medical morality to bind all who profess to heal. The philosophical justifications for medical morality are, I believe, appropriate but not sufficient for the Christian physician.

A refurbished medical morality taught in secular medical schools would provide Christian medical teachers and students with a starting point. Beyond that, they would depend on their own formation as Christians, on the assistance and counseling of Christian faculty members and on the support of the campus ministry. Formation of associations of Christian faculty and medical students in secular medical schools is a necessity, and is now a reality in a number of such schools.

Christian faculty members teaching in secular institutions have a heavy obligation and a special ministry. They must meet the special teaching needs of Christian medical students, practicing the Christian healing ministry for the edification of nonbelievers and members of non-Christian religious congregations as well. The task for Christian faculty members in secular institutions is difficult and demanding but also most rewarding as I have experienced it in most of my own teaching career.

The Christian medical student in a secular medical school also has special obligations. He or she must be a witness to Christianity, seek his or her own spiritual development, do extra reading in ethics, theology and philosophy, and work with other Christians to clarify and deepen their idea of what it means to be both a Christian and a physician. It is not enough to be first one and then the other. What is demanded of all—faculty, students and institutions—is the fusion in the fire of faith and reason of the two existential states of being a physician and being a Christian, a fusion so perfect that we cannot separate curing and healing from ministry and faith.

Christians are different because they are redeemed by Jesus Christ. As the Jews were freed from slavery to Pharaoh, Christians have been freed to enjoy the spiritual fullness of Christian service.

Christ's act of redemption imposes a higher morality than human reason alone can devise. Those higher moral duties transform the "practice of medicine" into a "ministry of healing." Christian medical students, teachers and practitioners are called to teach those duties to each other by example and precept.

I would like to close with a quotation from Father Thomas Merton, the Cistercian monk who reached out from the solitude of his monastery to engage the most crucial issues of our day: "The Christian is, I believe, one who abandons an incomplete life for a life that is integral, unified and structurally perfect. Yet this entrance into such a life is not the end of the journey but only the beginning."[13]

Notes

[1]Examples of this fusion of healing and ministry in Christ's life are too familiar to document. In Mark alone, there are some twenty instances. One of the most vivid is the following: "That evening, at sundown, they brought to him all who were sick or possessed with demons. And the whole city was gathered together about the door. And he healed many who were sick with various diseases, and cast out many demons; and he would not permit the demons to speak, because they knew him" (Mk. 1:32-34).

[2]E. D. Pellegrino, "Educating the Humanist Physician: An Ancient Ideal Reconsidered," *Journal of the American Medical Association*, 222, No. 11 March 1974), 1288-94.

[3]This transformation is evident if we compare the detailed presentations of medical morality in the first AMA code in 1848 and the recently proposed revisions. (Bruce Nortell, "AMA Judicial Activities," *Journal of the American Medical Association*, 239, No. 14 [3 April 1978], 1396-97.) The most recent versions are spare, noncommittal documents, like the testimony of a practiced witness in court who offers a minimum of comment to avoid further inquiry.

[4]E. D. Pellegrino, "The Fact of Illness and the Act of Pro-fession: Some Notes on the Source of Professional Obligation," in *Implications of History and Ethics to Medicine, Veterinary and Human*, ed. Laurence B. McCullough and James Polk Morris III, Centennial Academic Assembly (College Station, Tex.: Texas A & M, 1978), pp. 78-89.

[5]E. D. Pellegrino, "The Anatomy of Clinical Judgments," to appear in Vol. VI, *Philosophy and Medicine* (Dordrecht, The Netherlands: D. Reidel). See also Pellegrino, "The Fact of Illness."

[6]Ibid.

[7]I have drawn on the excellent William Osler Oration in the History of Medicine, "The Professional Ethics of the Greek Physician," in L. Edelstein, *Ancient Medicine*, eds. Owsei Temkin and C. Lillian Temkin (Baltimore: The Johns Hopkins Press, 1967), pp. 319-48.

[8]Scribonius Largus, *Compositions*, ed. Georgius Helmreich (Lipsiae, 1889).

[9]I refer here to almost a decade of experience that we in the Institute of Human Values in Medicine have gained with the teaching of the humanities in medical schools. These experiences are detailed in the reports of the Institute for Human Values, Witherspoon Building, Philadelphia, Pa.

[10]John Henry Newman, *On the Scope and Nature of University Education*, Introduction by Wilfred Ward, Prefatory Notes by Herbert Keldany (Dutton, N.Y.: Everyman's Library, 1965), p. 54.

[11]E. D. Pellegrino, "The Catholic Hospital: Options for Survival," *Hospital Progress*, 56, No. 2 (February 1975).

[12]E. D. Pellegrino, "Philosophy and Ethics of Medical Education," *The Encyclopedia of Bioethics*, ed. Warren T. Reich (Riverside, N.J.: Free Press [Macmillan], 1978).

[13]"The Monastic Journey," *A Thomas Merton Reader*, ed. Patrick Hart (New York: Doubleday Image Books, 1978), p. 12.

Part III

Models of Whole-Person Medicine

Chapter Seven

A Biblical Basis for Whole-Person Health Care: Theoretical and Practical Models in Health and Healing

James F. Jekel

In 1962 Thomas Kuhn published his now famous book *The Structure of Scientific Revolutions*, in which he debated the logical positivist idea that science progresses gradually from one stage to the next strictly on the basis of reason.[1] Kuhn argued that science progresses from one stage to another through intellectually and emotionally turbulent periods of conceptual revolution; these revolutions are followed by extended eras of relative quiet, during which the scientific field seeks to re-examine its subject matter from new perspectives with new assumptions acquired during the revolution. Kuhn called the new synthesis a *paradigm*. One quiet period continues until the assumptions and methods of the reigning paradigm prove insufficient to answer the new questions that appear. Thus, according to Kuhn, the progress of science is more like climbing uneven stairs than riding up a smooth ramp.

In the area of health care we are now entering a period of conceptual revolution which bears similarity to those described by Kuhn. The assumptions and methods of current medical research and care are increasingly being subjected to intense debate, which will lead to a different synthesis or paradigm, probably within the next decade or two. The ORU conference is evidence of the debate over the currently reigning "biomedical paradigm." We are among those searching for a more satisfactory paradigm than the one which now reigns supreme. The next paradigm, or model, of reality will undoubtedly contain most elements of the current biomedical model but will add other dimensions largely ignored by biomedicine.

For the most part, the added dimensions (social, psychological and spiritual) are given lip service and have been considered for a long time to be part of good medical care. Often, however, perhaps usually, they are ignored in the practice of medicine and in medical research. Good whole-person medicine is neither antiscientific nor will it ignore good science. It will, however, insist that all dimensions of human life be considered in medical research. Indeed, if whole-person medicine is to become the mainstream of health care, it will have to build a strong research base; without such a foundation, the existing medical educational institutions are not likely to be convinced that they should modify current emphases. It is important to distinguish "whole-person medicine" as a concept and as an approach to care from the "holistic medicine" movement with its many elements of Eastern mysticism, such as astrology. "Holistic medicine" is in danger of discrediting the legitimate concerns of this conference in the eyes of the scientific community. The distinction must be kept clear.

Many groups concerned to amplify the biomedical model, but without sharing the biblically based theism of this conference, use terms such as "holistic" medicine. Therefore, even among those who agree that biomedicine has failed to address the whole problem or the whole person, considerable disagreement exists as to what constitutes the whole. I would surmise that we are in general agreement that, in addition to the anatomic and biochemical dimensions, the whole person has psychological, social, and religious and spiritual dimensions, and that all of these must be accounted for in an adequate understanding of health, disease and healing. To consider all of these dimensions in the clinical setting, at one point in time, may be considered cross-sectional adequacy. Part of the current complaint against biomedicine, however, is that even within the biomedical realm the prophets of the current model have failed to give adequate attention to longitudinal adequacy, that is, to (1) a proper understanding of the historical roots of anatomic and physiologic distortions, (2) an epidemiologic approach to the natural history of disease and (3) a proper use of biomedical knowledge for care when cure is not possible.

Let us not assume that it will be easy to achieve a major change in the current biomedical paradigm. Despite the numerous and increasingly strident calls for change, the current biomedical paradigm's assumptions and methods are deeply entrenched at every level of our society, not just in medicine. The forces defending that paradigm are extremely powerful in scientific, economic and political influence. Moreover, the health-care system is now the nation's largest employer, with representatives in almost every community in the country, which means that there is a large constituency available to fight for the status quo.

Past and Present Contributions of Medicine
The current medical paradigm is not so sharply delineated as was, for example, the geocentric view of the universe or Newtonian physics. Nevertheless, many of its assumptions may be summarized. First, it assumes that our current level of health is due mainly to our public-health/medical-care system, which began with the development of the germ theory in the later 1800s. It is a popular idea that the control of communicable disease is largely the achievement of medical science (through immunization, antibiotics and so on). Historians, however, have increasingly come to understand that medicine as it has been practiced during the past century has had relatively little impact in producing the level of health we enjoy today.[2]

The sanitary revolution in Europe, particularly in England, was well underway, and its impact in reducing infant mortality was already being seen, before the development of the germ theory. The sanitary revolution came about from many people's personal convictions, which were partly biblical in origin, that it was better for society's health and morals to live in cleanliness than in filth. The germ theory reinforced that movement, of course, and strengthened its theoretical foundations, but was not its cause. Yet it was the sanitary revolution which, as much as any other factor, has restored society to today's levels of health. The term *restored* is at least partly correct here, because many of the infectious diseases—including the leading killers, tuberculosis and infant diarrhea—were made much more severe by the processes of urbanization and industrialization. Their resolution over the past century has been primarily a process of learning to live in industrial cities without opening the floodgate to disease.

Tuberculosis, for example, was the leading killer in the industrial West in the mid-1800s, with death rates that sometimes exceeded 500 per 100,000 per year. The death rates of tuberculosis have been declining steadily since about 1850. By 1949 it had become only a shadow of its former self, although medicine had no effective cure (that could significantly affect the death rate) before 1949, when streptomycin was discovered. Tuberculosis declined, not because of scientific medicine, but because of a number of related social and technical changes that were largely outside the purview of medicine, such as: improvement in nutrition, socioeconomic status and living and working conditions (especially the reduction of crowding); elimination of the spread of some tuberculosis through milk by pasteurization and elimination of infected herds; and increased genetic resistance of the population to the disease.

Most of the epidemic infectious diseases were also declining rapidly during the late 1800s and early 1900s, before medicine had either immunization (except for smallpox) or antibiotics. The world-renowned bacteriologist from the Rockefeller Foundation, René Dubos, put it this way:

> Clearly, modern medical science has helped to clean up the mess created by urban and industrial civilization. However, by the time laboratory medicine came effectively into the picture the job had been carried far toward completion by the humanitarians and social reformers of the nineteenth

century. Their romantic doctrine that nature is holy and healthful was scientifically naive but proved highly effective in dealing with the most important health problems of their age. When the tide is receding from the beach it is easy to have the illusion that one can empty the ocean by removing water with a pail. The tide of infectious and nutritional diseases was rapidly receding when the laboratory scientist moved into action at the end of the past century.[3]
The past president of the Blue Cross Association, Walter J. McNerney, listed as the first health myth to be debunked the idea that "most health services make a big difference in the health of a population, thus, with enough money, health can be purchased."[4] Even an apologist for modern biomedical technology, Lewis Thomas, has said: "In any case, we do not really owe much of today's population problems to the technology of medicine. . . . Modern medical science is a recent arrival, and the world population had already been set on what seems to be its irreversible course by the civilizing technologies of agriculture, engineering, and sanitation,—most especially the latter."[5]

Life Expectancy
A second doubtful assumption is that medical science will give us very long life spans. Because our life expectancy *at birth* has increased approximately thirty years over the past century, it is assumed that biomedical technology will continue such progress into the future, so that in another century or so, our life expectancy may be a hundred years or so. That overlooks the fact that during the same past century, the life expectancy of white males at retirement age (65) has increased but a few years. Life expectancy at birth has improved greatly because of the reduction of infant mortality, childhood diseases, tuberculosis and so on. Most infants can now expect to reach retirement age. What has not happened is a major change in the maximum length of life, since modern medical science has little capacity to alter significantly the course of the chronic degenerative diseases. It is as true now as when Moses wrote the ninetieth psalm (approximately 1400 B.C.) that

"the days of our years are threescore years and ten; and if by reason of strength they be fourscore . . ." (Ps. 90:10 KJV).

As Lewis Thomas says, "If we are not struck down prematurely by one or another of today's diseases, we live a certain length of time and then we die, and I doubt that medicine will ever gain a capacity to do anything much to modify this. I can see no reason for trying and no hope of success anyway. At a certain age, it is in our nature to wear out, to come unhinged and to die, and that is that."[6] He does add a salutary emphasis on the quality, rather than the quantity of life, which is certainly consistent with the biblical perspective: "My point here is that I very much doubt that the age at which this happens will be very drastically changed, for most of us, when we have learned more about how to control disease. The main difference will be that many of us will die in relatively good health."[7]

Although there will undoubtedly be some further progress toward increasing life expectancy, society must not look to scientific medicine to bring us eternal life.

The Biomedical Model

The underlying assumption of modern medicine and health care is what many have called the biomedical model. This model assumes that our lack of health is primarily due to *disease,* that most of our diseases are associated with anatomic and physiologic changes, and that diseases can be cured if such alterations are restored to their normal state. Disease is seen fundamentally as alterations in body anatomy and physiology, usually in predictable patterns. The task of the scientist and physician is to identify the abnormalities associated with the disease and discover methods of restoring these to "normal," which is seen as being equivalent to a "cure."

The largest institution built in honor of this assumption is the National Institutes of Health, which was expanded in 1948 and which has guided the direction of American medical research and (hence) medical education and practice since the early 1950s. Great achievements have been made in many dimensions of our knowledge of disease, but great problems have also been produced. Medicine has rapidly become more complex and dependent on expensive diagnostic and therapeutic technology. In turn, that has fostered specialization and other expensive changes. Legal and ethical problems are created faster than they are solved. The human dimension is being lost from the medical-care process.[8]

Medical education has almost lost sight of an increasingly well-documented fact, namely, nutrition, environment and behavior contribute heavily to the origin of most of our diseases. As George Engel has put it, "In modern Western society biomedicine not only has provided a basis for the scientific study of disease, it has also become our own culturally specific perspective about disease, that is, *our folk model* [italics mine]. Indeed, the biomedical model is now the dominant folk model of disease in the Western World."[9]

Engel suggests that a new paradigm should be based on a biopsychosocial model in which the role of social and psychological factors is adequately emphasized. I would like to add the spiritual dimension to his list. I believe that sooner or later we will discover that we cannot adequately deal with the subject of disease, and even less with the idea of health, without considering the meaning and purpose of life, and an individual's relationship to the Creator. Thanatology is one modern area of specialization which is gradually appreciating this truth.

One of the weaknesses of the biomedical model is its lack of concern with health and its inability to deal with it. We have more than one hundred schools of disease in this country, but few, if any, schools of health. Medical schools notoriously focus most of their effort on teaching about disease, especially its diagnosis and treatment. Schools of public health emphasize the origin of disease and the organization of care, rather than how to promote health. But, as the World Health Organization's preamble states, "Health is ... not merely the absence of disease or infirmity." We must face realistically the fact that we do not have a "health-care system." We have a "disease-care system" in which little effort is made to promote health in a positive sense.

Definition of Health

As a matter of fact, one of the difficulties we have in setting national health goals and measuring our progress (or lack of it) is our inability to define health with sufficient specificity to guide progress or evaluate impact. The WHO statement just quoted defines health as "a state of complete physical, mental, and social well-being. . . , " which, in addition to specifying a state unattainable in this life, is not very helpful. Dubos has pointed to one weakness of the biomedical model: "Health and disease cannot be defined merely in terms of anatomical, physiological, or mental attributes. Their real measure is the ability of the individual to function in a manner acceptable to himself and to the group of which he is a part."[10]

Thus, social functioning, not biochemical state, may be closer to a useful concept of health, and may also be easier to measure. It is not so widely accepted to date, partly because it has ambiguities and partly because to agree on such a definition would open the floodgates to a reallocation of resources away from what are now considered health activities.

Dubos and others have emphasized that health is not so much freedom from stress (which is unattainable in our sinful world) as it is the ability to adapt to the stresses to which we are subject: "The states of health or disease are the expressions of the success or failure experienced by the organism in its efforts to respond adaptively to environmental challenges."[11]

Rates of death and illness are clearly insufficient to measure health; at most they measure some of the deviations from it. In the last analysis, one must agree with Duncan Clark that "As for health. . . , no fully acceptable concept exists."[12] Here is certainly a fruitful field of research for those with a biblical perspective.

Iatrogenesis

In my first contact with Carl Moyer, our professor of surgery, he began his lecture with the Latin phrase, *primum non nocere*, which I understand can be translated "first, do not harm." It is a principle that made sense at that time (1958) and makes even more sense today. The first obligation of a physician should be not to harm the patient. It would also seem reasonable that the first obligation of the health-care *system* should be to do no harm.

Yet there is evidence that the medical-care system does a great deal of harm to individuals, through unnecessary surgery, through inappropriate or unnecessary medications and through pointing to pharmacologic or surgical solutions when changes in environment, lifestyle or human relationships are the only remedies that offer hope for real improvement. Much of the unnecessary surgery that is done stems from economic pressures in cities with more surgeons than are needed, and it is reinforced by the population's tendency to look to surgeons as modern miracle workers. Overmedication may arise from a sense of despair on the physician's part ("I don't know what else to do") or from the need to get on to the next patient. One study showed that physicians often write prescriptions for medication as a ritualistic way of terminating a patient visit, even in the absence of a clear indication for the medication.

Less studied but perhaps more important sources of harm from our medical-care approach are certain effects of a strongly institutionalized biomedical model of health and healing. Ivan Illich calls those effects "social and cultural iatrogenesis"; they are social and cultural distortions that occur by strict adherence to the biomedical model of disease.[13] I. K. Zola also points to social dangers inherent in the increasing medicalization of life.[14] We are turning less to religion or law, and more to medicine, for the final decision in social problems. Thus behavior (for example, murder) which centuries ago might have been dealt with as a problem of sin and more recently as lawlessness, now is first subjected to a medical test: if the perpetrator was somehow "ill" at the time of the act, he becomes "not guilty by reason of insanity." The point here is not to argue whether that is good or bad, but to emphasize that the final tribunal, and the first agent of attempted change, in this, as in countless other areas of life, is coming to be medical authority.

The medicalization of life also increases the *social control* which a small group of persons (health professionals) exercises over others. Thus, as a society, we have given to the physician the ultimate right to decide who does and does not have access to large amounts of society's resources. A decision to give someone a heart transplant, or to put someone on renal dialysis, may cost society $50,000 or more. The decision to give one person such resources means that others will not have access to them, because society's resources are limited.

Further, society has given the physician the power to give to some and to withhold from others the right to a socially acceptable form of deviance known as sickness. Talcott Parsons first clearly defined the social contract of Western society known as the "sick role," in which society gives certain benefits to a person defined by a "competent professional" as ill and requires certain behavior from that person. Society offers a sick person two advantages: freedom from blame for his or her condition and excuse from normal role obligations during the illness. In return society requires the individual: first, to want to recover and to seek out competent medical help, and second, to cooperate with those who are prescribing the therapy. Sociologists are increasingly concerned over the power given to the medical profession.

Costs
It is the cost of our current direction in medical care that will ultimately force major changes in the way we approach health care. The society will no longer tolerate an inflation in the cost of medical care that is twice the national average, when we are already spending about 9 per cent of the gross national product on medical care. We hear stories such as that General Motors now pays more to Blue Cross and Blue Shield than to U. S. Steel in a given year. That might be all right if we were getting a proportional benefit, but increasingly the population is becoming restless and is questioning whether it is receiving its money's worth. Certainly the marvels continue for many forms of acute medical problems and accidents. But as the population now is mostly living past retirement age, a

higher and higher proportion of all care is for chronic problems, where the biomedical approach has the least effect.

Lewis Thomas has this to say about the application of inadequate technology: "Offhand, I cannot think of any important human disease for which medicine possesses the capacity to prevent or cure outright where the cost of the technology is itself a major problem. The price is never as high as the cost of managing the same diseases during the earlier stages of ineffective technology."[15] Most examples of "effective technology" relate either to infectious disease or to acute medical and surgical emergencies. We should not deny the individual contributions of modern medicine in these areas; we should be grateful. What is of concern is that modern medicine, which can be so effective in restoring individuals with certain kinds of problems to productive life, is now becoming so saddled with ineffective technology in other areas that its real contributions are becoming less available to the average person. It is especially unlikely that our expensive Western medical technology, complete with its folk model of disease, can benefit the developing nations, even though we are exporting it at this time, in part through medical missions.

A new approach to health and health care is clearly needed. What insights do the Scriptures provide about changes we should make in our assumptions, concepts and approaches?

Prevention as the Way to Health
Many biblical insights can be brought to a consideration of health. Foremost among them is that health is the result of a way of life and not the product of nostrums. The broad commands of Scripture portray God's will for his people: "Ye shall be holy: for I the LORD your God am holy" (Lev. 19:2 KJV). The holy walk with God emphasized not defiling oneself (Lev. 11:44), which required, among other things, that a person distinguish "between holy and unholy, and between unclean and clean" (Lev. 10:10 KJV). The Scriptures provided the guidelines, and obedience carried the promise of physical blessings (health as well as spiritual blessings): "If you will diligently hearken to the voice of the LORD your God, and

do that which is right in his eyes, and give heed to his commandments and keep all his statutes, I will put none of the diseases upon you which I put upon the Egyptians; for I am the LORD, your healer" (Ex. 15:26).

At the pool of Bethesda, Jesus healed a man who had been ill for thirty-eight years and told him, "Sin no more, that nothing worse befall you" (Jn. 5:14). In Leviticus 18:5, God tells his people through Moses, "You shall therefore keep my statutes and my ordinances, by doing which a man shall live." Other Scriptures could be quoted, but the main point is that the biblical view of health is something that was a result of one's entire way of life, *not a commodity that could be purchased from healers*. Health included the idea of wholeness, soundness, safety and peace. Our world desperately needs to get away from the idea of health as a commodity, a product, and to see it as an organic part of one's way of life.

Many specific elements related to good health can be identified by epidemiology, the science of determining why disease (or health) occur when they do and in whom they do.

Nutrition
Fundamental to good health is nutrition. Malnutrition can be either undernutrition or overnutrition. By and large, undernutrition is the plight of the poor wherever they are in the world, and overnutrition is the companion of the well-to-do. Undernutrition not only robs one of the vigor to be creative and productive, but protein undernutrition, in particular, also combines synergistically with the infectious diseases to produce high mortality rates among children, particularly following the period of weaning. For example, measles is a serious but seldom fatal illness among unimmunized but well-nourished children, but it can have case fatality rates as high as 20 or 25 per cent among malnourished children, a death rate hundreds of times as high as among well-nourished children.[16] On the other hand, overnutrition, particularly when combined with a sedentary lifestyle, contributes to a variety of degenerative disorders in adults, such as coronary artery disease, strokes and diabetes. For example, the dietary intake

of refined sugar (sucrose) in this country in 1850 was about forty pounds per person per year; now it is over one hundred pounds per person per year.

Environment

A second foundation of health is a clean environment. Although that includes cleanliness from the many microbes capable of causing severe disease in humans, it does not imply a sterile existence. The importance of cleanliness was demonstrated during the sanitary revolution. Clean water, food and living environment are all important. Recently we have become more aware of the problem of toxic substances in water, food and the air, but at present we have only hints as to how such pollution may affect human health.

Behavior

Central to a way of life is one's behavior. Every aspect of our behavior has health implications, although often we do not realize it. Most Americans who smoke are aware of the potential risks that smoking brings for cancer of the bronchus, throat, nose and mouth. Less well known is that cigarette smoking also increases risk for heart attacks. Behavioral impact on health may be very subtle. For example, the Islamic custom of *purdah,* by keeping the women from sunlight, may reduce the available vitamin D and lead to osteomalacia in adolescent women. In turn, that frequently produces deformed pelves and difficult labor and delivery, causing infant and maternal mortality.

In many developing nations, women seek to wean children early and convert to bottle feeding in order to imitate the wealthy. Because of lack of refrigeration, the milk is likely to be swarming with bacteria, and because of the low purchasing power of poor families, the "milk" may be only water colored with a small amount of powdered milk.[17] It is not known how much malnutrition among young children results from early weaning from the breast to the bottle, but the toll is probably heavy. Moreover, by shortening the nursing period, women reach peak fecundity sooner following the delivery of a child than they would if they nursed over a longer time, and thus the same behavior pattern also contributes to increased worldwide fertility.[18]

The venereal diseases are among the commonest types of infectious disease in the West. Estimates of the number of new cases of gonorrhea in 1978 went over two million. Syphilis, although not rampant, remains steady at approximately 100,000 per year in the United States. A newly appreciated venereal threat is from herpes viruses, especially HVH II. Antibiotics have proved impotent to eradicate these diseases; control of behavior could eradicate them.

The above three factors—nutrition, environment and behavior—are primary factors influencing the level of health any population enjoys. Medical care is at most the "fine tuning" of our health level; the other factors determine the "channel." It is instructive to review the biblical concern for human nutrition, sanitation and behavior. Concern for proper and pure food is seen in many biblical references (see Figure 7.1). Concern for personal cleanliness, pure water, sewage disposal, rapid burial of the dead and isolation from contamination by discharges is quite specific. Behavior was carefully prescribed both as to justice and as to cleanliness, and venereal disease was effectively prevented by the code of sexual morality (Ex. 20:14; Lev. 18:20 and elsewhere). Moreover, the priest served as the health officer, to oversee that the community was holy and clean, to diagnose and treat problems and to pronounce healed persons clean (Lev. 13—14). More important than specific commands is the totality of the pattern of prevention and its integration into a way of life with a spiritual foundation.

In summary, the biblical insight that health derives from a holy and clean way of life, and not from purchasing the services of healers, is a perspective our society must recover if we are to achieve the measure of health we desire, at a price we can afford. But who can influence human behavior? How we behave derives from what we ultimately believe is of greatest value. In determining the priorities of individuals, families and communities, religion has a crucial impact on health.

Figure 7.1 The Sanitary Code in the Old Testament (Selections)

Key Texts: Leviticus 19:2; 10:10

1. *Personal Cleanliness*
   Hand washing, especially before meals *Mark 7:1-3*
   Washing whole body after contamination *Leviticus 15:5*
   Washing clothes after contamination *Leviticus 11:28; 15:5*

2. *Pure Water Supply*
   Avoid water contaminated by dead animal *Leviticus 11:32-36*

3. *Sewage Disposal*
   Bury wastes outside the camp *Deuteronomy 23:12-14*

4. *Early Burial*
   Interment before nightfall *Deuteronomy 21:23; Acts 5:6*

5. *Pure Foods*
   Fruits and vegetables not prohibited
   Meats *Leviticus 11:1-8, 29-31*
   Fish *Leviticus 11:9-12*
   Don't eat dead animals *Deuteronomy 14:21*
   Don't eat old food *Leviticus 19:5-8*

6. *Isolation*
   If one touches the dead *Leviticus 5:2; 22:4*
   If one touches unclean discharges *Leviticus 5:3*
   For those who have a discharge *Leviticus 15:1-13*
   For those who have skin diseases *Leviticus 13*
   Of a woman following childbirth *Leviticus 12:1-8*
   (prevents epidemic "childbed fever")
   Terminal disinfection *Leviticus 15:1-13; 14:34-48*

7. *Control of Venereal Disease*
   Morality *Exodus 20:14; Leviticus 18:20*

8. *Priest as Health Officer*
   Leviticus 13–14

Summary: Health consists of walking in a right relationship to a holy God. This walk must be a holy walk. Thus cleanliness is required for every aspect of life, and one must be constantly seeking the clean and holy way. Health, then, is not to be found in nostrums, but rather in the cleansing of body and spirit (Lev. 15:13-15) and in a holy way of life (see key texts above).

Quantity or Quality of Life?

Only in recent years has any serious challenge been raised to the priorities of medical care; heretofore, the first priority has been to save (or prolong) life, regardless of the cost in money and suffering. Death rates are the best developed and most used measure of the success or failure of our medical-care system. Development of the technology of medicine to include organ transplants, artificial life-support systems and so on has forced reconsideration of the limits of medicine with respect to prolonging life. For a time there was a lot of talk of "cryogenics," in which bodies would be frozen immediately at death and kept in deep freeze, along with all medical records, until medical science discovered a way to thaw the body, revive it and, simultaneously, cure the disease.

Increasingly, people agree that saving lives is an appropriate first priority in acute disease, but that improving the quality of life is a more appropriate and realistic goal than extreme efforts to prolong life in chronic, degenerative diseases. Even a leading proponent of biomedical technology seems to be saying the same thing.[19] The problem is that although lip service is paid to the idea of retooling the delivery of care to emphasize the quality of life, such priorities are seldom reflected in the objectives of current medical research and education. Nutrition is a neglected subject in our schools of medicine and public health. So is rehabilitation. "Cure" is taught much better than "care." But for a number of reasons, including economic ones, new kinds of primary-care professionals are being trained (for example, nurse-practitioners and physicians' assistants) who often have a better grasp of the meaning of care than physicians. The cost of hospital care is forcing an expansion of home-care programs. People are finding that alternatives such as the hospice are better for persons dying of cancer than the typical acute hospital.[20] The coming revolution in medical care will move the "quality of life" to a new place of prominence in the priorities of medical care.

The biblical message is concerned for both the quantity and quality of human life. Yet those are not primary goals; rather they are the result of obedience to God as revealed in the Scriptures. Biblical concern for faith, obedience, holiness and justice clearly places those who stand in the Hebrew-Christian tradition in the position of supporting a balance. We should vigorously support efforts to restore concern for the quality of life to its rightful position in medical care. Moreover, as one considers the nature of health, it is important to see that the healthy person is one for whom life, with all of its activities, has deep personal meaning.

At the level of tactics, Viktor Frankl has demonstrated how important it is for life to have meaning.[21] He gives an example of how an elderly man was restored to mental health when he saw that surviving his wife and the resultant loneliness meant that his beloved wife did not have to suffer the same; his suffering then had meaning for him and became a last sacrifice for her. Only then was it tolerable. Going further, it yet remains for someone to demonstrate that human wholeness—health if you will—must include our ability to stand before God as justified sinners. There are suggestions that those who wholeheartedly embrace the full theological meaning of the Bible are better able to live, and to die, in health. That area needs far more research.

Setting for Healing: The Family's Role

One myth about medical care is that most medical care is given by health professionals. Levin and others have emphasized that, in fact, perhaps 75 per cent of all health care in this country is given by individuals to themselves or to members of their families.[22] It is as foolish to see that as bad as it is to consider all professional care good. There is currently a powerful movement, often called the self-care movement, to increase the competence of nonprofessionals to care for themselves and others. Its emphasis is not that "kitchen surgery" should return, but rather that all efforts should be made to give the individual person and family as much responsibility over their own lives and health as possible. The role of the physician will increasingly become (1) to do the highly technical, advanced diagnosis and treatment, and (2) to serve as consultant to those giving most of the health care: families and nonphysician primary-care persons. We cannot afford to restore physicians to their past prominent role as givers of primary care; they are too costly, and they are not trained well for that task anyway.

Norman Cousins gave a dazzling account of his determination to treat himself for a condition considered medically hopeless and of his success.[23]

A prominent sociologist, Lois Pratt, points out:

The more numerous and vital the functions the family performs successfully for its members, the stronger is the family system; the fewer the important functions performed, the weaker the system. . . . The family is a social unit with considerable potential for performing health care, since families are held legally responsible for sustaining their members' health; they maintain a physical plant which is suitable for health-care practice, and the members live together in relationships of mutual care and support.[24]

She reminds us of current trends, which are in contrast with the potential of the family to perform health care:

The emerging medical-care system is based on specialization of work, centralization of activity in large complex units, bureaucratization of the work unit, control by management over work and personnel, corporate involvement in and exploitation of all aspects of the health market, and extension of profit-making to all sectors of health care.[25]

One byproduct of the large health institutions we are creating is impersonal care. How can costs be reduced and care be as personal as possible? By restoring care to the context of a loving family. The medical-care system should be, in the last analysis, a family support system, or so it seems to me. At present, however, families do a better job of supporting the health system (most persons in health care are doing well economically) than the system is doing of supporting the family (office and clinic hours are for the convenience of the provider rather than the patient, as are appointments, and so on). The emergency room has gained immense popularity, not because it is the best place to receive care, but because it is the only place people know will be open twenty-four hours a day with someone there to see them.

Whether or not the self-care movement will be sustained, its existence has shown that there are options available to the family. The family should play an increased role in the future in (1) selecting, coordinating and supervising professional care; (2) determining the forms and conditions of medical intervention; (3) evaluating the outcomes of all those interventions; (4) maintaining health records on the family; and (5) planning a healthy lifestyle, including the choice of community, residence, employment, leisure activity, diet and other health maintenance practices. Certainly not all families or individuals now either want that role or are capable of it. But in that direction may lie our best hope for both economy and effectiveness of health care.

The Bible does not appear, at first glance, to inject itself into this debate. But on further consideration it seems to suggest that healing is, in fact, the proper role for the family, including the larger family of a religious congregation. The fifth commandment (honor thy father and mother) is often interpreted as applying only to young children and their parents. Jesus, however, interpreted it as caring for one's aged parents (Mk. 7:10-13). If interpreted in that way, the promise (long life) has special meaning. In Acts 6 and James 1 there are evidences that the early church received and acted on the command to care for each other; James 5:14 shows that a healing ministry was included. (The oil in that passage should probably be seen as having medicinal value rather than spiritual significance; for example, note the use of oil in Lk. 10:34.) The pattern of individuals giving health care to each other in a family context seems to have solid scriptural support.

Haggerty is one of many whose studies have shown that persons under stress have a higher risk of disease. He suggests that clinicians can be more effective in preventing the harmful potentials of stress by drawing on supportive institutions beyond the primary family: the extended family, peer groups, religious groups. The assumption behind such a proposal is that human beings are social creatures who need complex and supportive interaction with groups. Without it, we get sick, just as an infant deprived of love tends to die.[26] We need social support in order to resist stress. Research appears to be indicating that in the presence of social supports, such as family and close friends, a given noxious stimulus is less likely to produce disease. As Cassel states: "these studies would suggest that at both the human and animal levels the presence of another particular animal of the same species may, under certain circumstances, protect the individual from a variety of stressful stimuli."[27]

Role of Family and Friends in Institutional Care

One principle of good care is that no institution for health care should isolate patients from their families nor fail to educate the patient and family to achieve the maximum self-care possible. As an extreme example, consider the regional perinatal centers in our country which, some believe, have contributed in recent years to lowering the infant mortality rate. Women may be separated from their home, family and community in order to enter a perinatal center, sometimes for several weeks, several hundred miles from home. What kind of disruption in family life is produced and what economic and emotional strains result? In the long run, are the benefits worth the cost to family relationships and integrity? Are there alternative ways to achieve the same good results that would support family integrity?

When the experience of childbirth was moved into hospitals there were unquestioned benefits to mothers and infants. But we have come to realize there were also costs other than dollars in the institutionalization of childbirth. The role of the husband, reduced to waiting-room isolation and agony, became a standard joke. The wife was isolated from her closest companion at a time when she needed emotional as well as medical support. Women made unconscious during delivery, and often during labor, lost the reality of an experience many cherish. Babies were largely kept from their mothers during the first twenty-four hours, a period which Klaus and others have shown to be important for the bonding of a mother to her infant.[28] Today efforts are made to include the family, as much as possible, in labor, delivery and aftercare, to enable "natural childbirth" to the extent desired and possible, and to have an alert mother and child with maximum interpersonal contact in the first twenty-four hours. The challenge here, as elsewhere, is to retain those aspects of medical excellence we now prize while restoring the experience, care and support to the family wherever possible.

What about classic hospital care for medical or surgical conditions? As mentioned earlier, the potentially dehumanizing aspects of such care have been extensively documented.[29] The Christian Medical Council, in its 1973 position paper, stated:

> The institutional environment itself often discriminates against the families most in need of support. The provision of health care, particularly in a prestigious hospital, may combine technical excellence with procedures which are destructive of family and social relationships. Ill health in itself places great strains on personal relationships, and the way that problems are handled can be healing in strengthening bonds of caring or grossly disruptive in callous unconcern for subtle relationships which form the fabric of life.

The paper concludes that one of the sources of injustice in health care arises because "the health care system does not promote the wholeness of individual, family and community life through its tendency to depersonalize individual care and disrupt interpersonal relationships, with those who suffer most often being those most in need."[30]

In our society, hospitalization forces almost total discontinuity with past and future existence. Every experience, and almost every person, is new and unfamiliar. Few patients are well prepared for hospitalization or for their discharge. I believe we could learn from some hospitals in tropical countries, where it is expected that the family will come and continue to care for the ill person. Individual hospital rooms are, in fact, areas where several family members can live, cook for and feed the patient, and give much of the nursing care.

That reduces costs greatly, puts responsibility for care where it belongs, on the family, and insures education of the family and continuity of care when the patient has returned home.

Why can't we learn from those examples? Why not make some U.S. hospital rooms with two (or even three) beds, only one of which would be equipped with oxygen and other patient needs. The other bed or beds (double-decker) would be for family members, who would live with the patient, order food from a menu appropriate to the patient's diet and feed the patient if necessary, give basic observation and nursing care and so on. Short-term education of family members in nursing techniques would surely be less costly than long-term care. The medical chart would be in the patient's room and the family would make appropriate care notes.[31] They would give medications and injections when feasible, regulate the flow of intravenous fluids and so on.

Such participation would not be for everyone, of course, either because some would not want it or because they could not work it out for reasons of health or other responsibilities. For those who could, however, and many families probably could for some illnesses and some times of the day, the family would protect the dignity and integrity of the loved one and would learn better how to assure continuity of care after discharge. Assisting in hospital care could be a tremendous area of service for the church. There is unexplored potential here to improve patient care while reducing costs and enhancing family competence, independence and relationships.

The challenge to Christians in giving wholistic care is to be daring and innovative, not just to put a thin veneer on existing patterns of care.[32] Unless the revolution in care is profound, it will not produce whole-person medicine.

Community-Wide Perspective

We want our medical institutions to be centers of excellence. One of the great misunderstandings of our day, however, is related to what makes an institution a "center of excellence." Lambourne described a pediatric hospital in Africa which was known to be a "center of excellence"; it was a source of great pride until someone studied trends in the infant mortality rate in the region the hospital served. Infant mortality was about 282 per 1000 live births, and had not changed very much over a decade. Appalled, the new director trained teenage women in how to diagnose and treat with medications three diseases: malaria (by history and feeling for the spleen), dysentery (by history and inspection of the stool) and sores (by history and inspection). Although the dispensers made mistakes, "in 5 years' time the infant mortality rate had dropped to 78/1000." That is just 28 per cent of what it had been before. Lambourne comments: "Now what was killing all those children before? A sacred, stereotyped view of excellence! That is, a graven image of excellence, tempting us to idolatry."[33]

In a similar vein, The Christian Medical Commission stated in a position paper:

> The primary requirement then is that there be no discrimination in the way we assume responsibility for total populations around our institutions. . . . First, instead of spending all our precious resources on those who come spontaneously, we must work out new ways of defining and providing a basic minimum of services for all. The definition of this basic minimum must be locally derived and strictly limited to ensure coverage. The second part of providing equitable distribution is to set and follow priorities in care.[34]

In my opinion, no center can be considered a center of excellence unless it is addressing effectively the needs of *all* people in the community it serves.

Toward an Applied Model of Whole-Person Medicine

An adequate conceptual model should help all participants in the healing effort: physicians, nurses, ministers, social workers, midlevel practitioners, family and others. Any model of healing must be based on an understanding of the causes of the problem. The *proximal* manifestations of disease, the anatomic and physiologic changes that accompany disease, are usually not the causes. They are better thought of as the "mechanisms" of a disease,[35] the causes of which lie farther back in history. There are *intermediate* causes (nutrition, environment, genes, behavior, and so on), and the *ultimate* cause, which according to Scripture is humanity's historical rebellion against its Creator. For example, to say that sin, malnutrition, obesity and biochemical abnormalities are all causes of diabetes mellitus is no more contradictory than to say that the cook, the oven and the heat baked the cake. The ultimate cause deals with *agency,* the intermediate cause with *sources,* and the proximal cause with the *mechanisms* of disease. A biblically adequate model must deal with all of those levels of causation (that is, it must be longitudinally adequate) if it is to promote health or to achieve a truly adequate healing.

I once treated a man for an unusual venereal disease. The disease itself responded to an antibiotic, because his biological healing powers were intact. But it was not his first episode of venereal disease; his marriage was on the rocks and he was seeking sexual expression elsewhere, yet he was miserable. To treat his biological problem without getting him and his wife into a therapeutic process to help his psychosocial problem was, in retrospect, inadequate healing. In his case, however, even marital counseling would have been inadequate unless someone had dealt with the spiritual problems, which, I sensed, both he and his wife had.

Modern biomedicine might say that the man was cured if the venereal disease organisms were no longer found in his body or that further healing was somebody else's responsibility. A modern advocate of wholistic medicine from agnostic assumptions might say that he was not healed until his marriage was restored to happiness. But to the Christian true healing would also mean that the couple be reconciled to their Creator.

Health as Reconciliation
I would like to suggest a concept of healing based on reconciliation. The word *reconciliation,* it is my hope, will convey sufficient and relatively unbiased meaning both to scientists and to theologians. The term implies restoration to harmony. Theologically the word is often found in the Scriptures.

Medically speaking, it implies removal of bad stressors (which produce dystress) and restoration to harmonious function. Here I use the term *stressor* to mean those noxious forces, agents or states (physical, biological, chemical, spiritual, social or psychological) which produce damage or force major adaptation by the individual. *Stress* means the nonspecific response of an organism to one or more stressors.[36] Not all stressors, and not all stress, are bad. In the form of, for example, infant stimulation, exposure to commensal microorganisms or exercise, stress is necessary for health and, indeed, for life. A moderate response to good stressors is called "eustress" by Selye.[37] Both types of stressor may come in oversupply and produce hyperstress, so that adaptation is difficult. Deficiency of all form of stressors produces hypostress.

Figure 7.2 shows a proposed model suggesting that health is a product of being fully (or at least adequately) reconciled on three dimensions: with the Creator, with other human beings, with the creation.[38] At each level, lack of reconciliation results in characteristic types of stressors and at each level specific types of reconciliation are needed in order to eliminate the stressors and promote health. Wholism here is seen in the reduction of all the bad stressors (lowering dystress) and restoration to harmonious functioning on three levels (eustress).

The model may be viewed as a kind of "review of systems" which could be used if one is to deal fully with a person's needs. Just as in a medical review of systems, in some areas no problems may emerge and in other areas the problems may not be particularly relevant to the chief complaint or need immediate attention. This is presented as a review of systems compatible with the biblical message and with both cross-sectional and longitudinal adequacy as defined above. It reviews the major areas with which whole-person medicine must be concerned.

As an example, the man I spoke of with the venereal disease needed: (1) an antibiotic (C-4 on Table 2); (2) a change in behavior and attitudes (C-3); reconciliation to fellowship with his wife (B-1); and, I believe, (4) forgiveness from the Creator

Figure 7.2 An Applied Model for Practitioners of Whole-Person Medicine, Based on the Concept of Health as Reconciliation in Three Dimensions

Reconciliation with:	Lack of Reconciliation Gives: (Dystress)	The Process of Reconciliation Gives: (Eustress)	Facilitators
A. The *Creator*	1. Guilt: spiritual, personal 2. Meaninglessness, lostness 3. Spiritual aloneness	1. Forgiveness (grace) 2. Life meaning and purpose 3. Knowledge of God's love	Theologians
B. Other *Persons*	1. Aloneness 2. Anomie 3. Powerlessness, helplessness	1. Fellowship with persons 2. Mediating structures[39] 3. Mutual support	Social Workers Family Church
C. The *Creation*	1. Malnutrition 2. Pollution 3. Unhealthful behavior 4. Anatomic & physiologic disruptions (alterations)	1. Good nutrition 2. Clean environment 3. Healthful behavior 4. Biomedical interventions	Physicians Nurses

and an altered sense of life purpose (A-1, 2).

Who is responsible for such healing? It is difficult and costly enough now to give care that is not wholistic. There are not enough primary practitioners currently to give adequate care to all, and this wholistic approach would, one would imagine, increase the load on primary care. However, as Lewis Thomas implied, healing with inadequate technology is very expensive, whereas healing with adequate technology is not. Restoring a patient to a right relationship to God, to home and community, and to the good earth will be, in the long run, less costly than care which is not wholistic and which is not true healing. Moreover, many others are equally important to the healing process, if physicians will relax their grip on the control of healing: ministers, nurses, midlevel practitioners, and—very crucial—family and friends, especially those of the church.

Note in Figure 7.2 that different professionals begin to work at different points in the review of systems. They may or may not move to different points in the model in any given patient contact. The *physician* begins with the anatomic and biochemical adjustments, and should, at least, make a diagnosis and give guidance concerning nutrition, behavior and so on. The *minister* begins at the opposite end and progresses toward the anatomic and biochemical adjustments (with which he or she will seldom deal). Physicians and theologians should both be concerned about social-psychological relationships in the middle of the model. On occasion a physician may be able to do more effective spiritual counseling than a minister, or a minister may be a more effective counselor than a physician with regard to lifestyle, nutrition or attitudes, and so on. A *social worker* would probably begin at the middle level (B) and work toward either end as indicated. The point is that no part of the systems review is totally out of the responsibility of any practitioner. Of course with surgery or prescriptions, nonphysicians may merely encourage compliance with medical suggestions.

The danger of overprofessionalization in the healing process (the idea that all healing must be referred to a pro-

fessional) is not new. Serious questions remain as to how far
and when each healer should use a full systems review. There
are questions regarding information divulgence and confi-
dentiality, and about who is "competent" to undertake such
a broad review. Considerable harm could come from charla-
tans or from well-meaning but inept practitioners trying a
wholistic systems review or treatment. Certain tests must be
passed before a patient is declared ready for open-heart
surgery—the same should be true before "open-soul surgery." What are the tests, and how does one know the correct
time to proceed with a full life-system review?

The patient may even need an ombudsman to act as his or
her advocate and defender within the system. The idea of
each patient (who so wishes) having both a physician and a
prayer-partner intrigues me; possibly the prayer-partner
could become the ombudsman in medical matters, the physician in spiritual matters. The prayer-partner could say to the
physician, "This patient is not emotionally and spiritually
ready for open-heart surgery"; the physician could say to the
prayer-partner, "This patient is not physically ready for open-
soul surgery." Each could serve as a corrective, a kind of
check and balance, to the other. Would such a practice potentially pit different professionals against each other where
disagreements arose? At times that may be preferable to one
specialist going on alone, unchecked. In medicine at least, we
constantly need to be reminded not to seize authority which
is properly the patient's or God's.

Of course, several professionals could find themselves in
agreement and "gang up" on the patient, being even more
intimidating than a single professional healer. The result
could be a patient even more dependent and passive than
when he or she had to deal with only one professional. In my
judgment, the corrective tendency will be far more frequent
and important. In any case, it is salutary to remind ourselves
that neither the physician nor other professionals actually do
the healing. That must be done by the patient and by the
Creator; the "healer," at most, makes conditions ideal for
healing to take place.

It is not clear to what extent reconciliation with the creation and with others can occur apart from reconciliation with the Creator. Certainly much helping and healing can occur for many people without direct reference to the spiritual dimension. It is my conviction, however, that healing (reconciliation) is always incomplete unless it includes the spiritual dimension.

I would like to conclude with a quotation from Canon Max Warren's book *The Christian Imperative:*

The fundamental sicknesses of men have always been sicknesses of the spirit and the mind. Never, perhaps, was this more obviously so than today.... Only a healing which makes a man whole and integrates him with his fellows in a true community, living in a right relationship with God and with the good earth which God has given man, only such a healing is adequate to the imperative "go heal." For this reason the Church must not imagine that it can relegate the responsibilities of its healing mission to a representative company of physicians and nurses, surgeons, and anesthetists, pathologists and dispensers....

The ... hospital must be seen as an integral part of a common task in which Church and school and farm are seen, not as the possibly attractive agencies for the employment of those with no skill in healing, but as the actual points at which most of the healing is done, the front line of the attack on human need. To these, the real centers of healing, the hospital will be related as a source of inspiration, a school of technical knowledge, a resort for such cases as demand specialized skill, but not as being itself the center of healing.[40]

Notes

[1]Nicholas Wade, "Thomas S. Kuhn: Revolutionary Theorist of Science," *Science,* 197 (8 July 1977), 143-45.

[2]Thomas McKeown, "Determinants of Health," *Human Nature,* 1, No. 4 (April 1978), 60-67.

[3]René Dubos, *Mirage of Health* (New York: Doubleday, 1961), pp. 30-31.

[4]Walter J. McNerney, "Health Care Reforms—The Myths and Realities,"

American Journal of Public Health, 61 (February 1971), 222-32.

[5]Lewis Thomas, "Aspects of Biomedical Science Policy," An Occasional Paper of the Institute of Medicine, National Academy of Sciences (1972), p. 10.

[6]Thomas, p. 9.

[7]Ibid.

[8]R. Duff and A. B. Hollingshead, *Sickness and Society* (New York: Harper & Row, 1968).

[9]George L. Engel, "The Need for a New Medical Model: A Challenge for Biomedicine," *Science,* 196 (8 April 1977), 129-36. The "folk model" includes ideas about the origin of disease (spontaneous), a healing class, the importance of medications, the centrality of cure and the inevitable progress of science.

[10]Dubos, *Mirage of Health,* p. 214.

[11]René Dubos, *Man Adapting* (New Haven, Conn.: Yale University Press, 1965), p. xvii.

[12]Duncan W. Clark, "A Vocabulary of Preventive Medicine," in *Preventive Medicine,* eds. Duncan W. Clark and B. MacMahon (New York: Little, Brown & Co., 1967), p. 3.

[13]Ivan Illich, *Medical Nemesis* (New York: Random House, 1976).

[14]I. K. Zola, "Medicine as an Institution of Social Control," in *A Sociology of Medical Practice,* eds. C. Cox and A. Mead (London: Collier-MacMillan, 1975).

[15]Lewis Thomas, p. 11.

[16]Nevin Scrimshaw, "Ecologic Factors Determining Nutritional State and Food Use," in *Alternatives for Balancing World Food Production Needs* (Ames, Iowa: Iowa State University Press, 1967), pp. 35-50.

[17]Ibid.

[18]Franz W. Rosa, "The Interaction of Breast Feeding and Family Planning in the Americas," mimeograph, n.d.

[19]Lewis Thomas, p. 9.

[20]J. Craven and F. Wald, "Hospice Care for Dying Patients," *American Journal of Nursing* (October 1975).

[21]Viktor Frankl, *Man's Search for Meaning* (New York: Washington Square Press, 1959).

[22]L. Levin, A. H. Katz and E. Holst, eds., *Self-Care: Lay Initiatives in Health* (New York: Prodist, 1976).

[23]Norman Cousins, "Anatomy of an Illness (As Perceived by the Patient)," *New England Journal of Medicine,* 295 (23 December 1976), 1458-63.

[24]Lois Pratt, "Changes in Health Care Ideology in Relation to Self-Care by Families," Paper presented at the annual meeting of the American Public Health Association, Miami Beach, Fla. (19 October 1976).

[25]Ibid.

[26]R. Haggerty, as reported in *Behavior Today,* 7, No. 42 (1 November 1976), 2.

[27]John Cassel, "Psychological Processes and Stress: Theoretical Formulation," *International Journal of Health Services,* 4, No. 3 (1974), 471-82.

[28]M. H. Klaus and J. H. Kennell, *Maternal Infant Bonding* (St. Louis: The C. V. Mosby Co., 1976).

[29]Duff and Hollingshead.

[30]Christian Medical Council, *Position Paper on Health Care and Justice*, Contact #16 (July 1973).

[31]The nursing station can be destructive to good patient care. There the doctor and nurses can hide behind charts and paperwork while patients are unattended or are seen by less-trained persons. Some hospitals, including one I have observed, have eliminated the nursing station for most wards. The patient's charts are in the room (unlocked), as are the medications (locked). The doctors and nurses must be in with the patients to do their tasks. Amazingly, the patients evidently receive more care.

[32]I am indebted to Marsha Fowler, R.N., M.S., for pointing out that many of the emphases in this paper about the understanding of disease and the provision of care are discussed and often applied within the nursing field. It is regrettable that medicine does not learn more from the nursing profession.

[33]R. A. Lambourne, "Secular and Christian Models of Health and Salvation," published as *Contact #1* by the Christian Medical Commission (November 1970).

[34]Christian Medical Council, *Position Paper.*

[35]From personal communication with Dr. A. M.-M. Payne, 1965.

[36]Cassel.

[37]Hans Selye, "How to Live with Stress," in *Help Yourself* (Chicago: Blue Cross Association, 1978).

[38]I am indebted to James Consedine, III for the suggestion that a fourth level of reconciliation be added to the model: reconciliation with one's self. For the present I have chosen not to include it, partly to keep the model as simple as possible. Also, the "self" is included in each of the other levels as the one who is reconciled to others. Moreover, the biblical perspective seems not to be introspective but rather outward-looking. This may be merely a matter of terminology: here "reconciliation" is used to indicate that a whole person is restored in his or her relationship to another. An individual person must be "integrated" (all dimensions functioning together harmoniously) for full reconciliation to be possible. I suspect, however, that the issue goes beyond terminology to anthropology: ultimately our interpretation of the meaning of whole-person care is dependent on our understanding of the nature and purpose of persons.

[39]I am indebted to Ian and Debra Kling for suggesting this term here. Examples of mediating structures are families, churches, voluntary associations and neighborhood organizations.

[40](New York: Charles Scribner's Sons, 1955), pp. 81-82.

Chapter Eight

Dissemination of Wholistic Health Centers

Granger E. Westberg

My education in the dissemination of wholistic health centers came in two stages. The first center was begun in a low-income neighborhood in 1970 in Springfield, Ohio, and was aimed at a population made up of 80 per cent Appalachian whites and 20 per cent blacks in a section of the city from which all doctors had moved. The emergency ambulance was frequently called into that section of the city, and other residents had to be taken by friends to the community hospital, about a mile and a half away, where they were seen in the emergency room. The local school nurse brought to our attention the great need for health care in that area.

The First Experiment
At that time I was teaching in the School of Theology at Wittenberg University and was experimenting with doing part of my teaching outside the seminary walls. I had a number of seminary students available to assist me in various projects related to the Good Shepherd Lutheran Church located in that low-income neighborhood. The nurse suggested that what we really needed was a doctor's office in the community. We decided to try to find physicians and nurses who would volunteer their services if we would set up a suitable location in the educational building of our church. After a lot of

searching, we found volunteer doctors and nurses. It was arranged that seminary students would take the social histories of patients and counsel with them. We then covered the area with brochures telling of the establishment of a doctor's office in a church, indicating that the service would be free to people living in the neighborhood. The school nurse had said that it was the sickest neighborhood in all of Springfield and was obviously the one most underserved. She was confident that patients would swarm into the building on the very first day it was open.

We opened on a Wednesday afternoon, all of us waiting for the crowd to arrive. Not a single patient came. So, we spent the next two weeks trying to sell residents on the new office by making personal calls in homes, speaking to the Parent-Teacher Association, and announcing it in the five local churches. We were open one Wednesday afternoon a week, but by the end of the third week we still had no patients. We decided to give it one more try. Finally our first patient came on the fourth Wednesday afternoon. She turned out to be a barmaid in a nearby tavern who came only because a neighbor had insisted that she come. She had been in bed for two days. Her visit to the clinic and her subsequent improvement marked the beginning of good public relations in the community because she had many friends. From then on the problem was not how to find enough patients but rather how to take care of the many patients beyond the daily thirty-patient limit.

The dissemination lesson we learned from that experience was that any project of this kind has to have the imprimatur of local people. They have to see it as fitting their needs and not just the needs of those operating the clinic. We learned later that people had hesitated to come because they were sure it was some kind of gimmick that the churches were using to get them to sit still to be preached at.

In other words, even though the need for medical care was obviously present in the community, resistance to the mode in which it was being offered slowed down its acceptance. Although free, it was still suspect. We also soon learned that we had to invite a number of volunteers from the neighborhood to participate in various forms in the wholistic health center. It gave credibility to the center to have neighbors there who could vouch for its quality of service.

The Springfield Center and another satellite center are still in operation even though the seminary students are no longer available because the seminary has moved to Columbus. We regret that the counseling aspect of the center's work has been greatly curtailed because of this loss of personnel. The physical side and some educational programs, however, are still in operation. Some of the original volunteers are giving hundreds of hours of service each year.

Another Environment

The dissemination problem in our second wholistic health center was similar in many respects although we were dealing with an entirely different population in an affluent community.

In 1972 I was invited to speak to a group of faculty and students at Howard University Medical School, Washington, D.C., concerning the possibility of starting a wholistic health center in that city. Their response to a doctor's office in a church with people to assist the physician in counseling and educational programs was very favorable, but they raised one major question: Are you only going to start centers in poor neighborhoods? They argued against this. One put it this way: "If you do this only in poor neighborhoods, you're going to give the impression that your kind of wholistic approach to health care is only for poor people. Clinics that start in poor neighborhoods are seen as giving second-rate medical care. Also, they seldom last more than a very few years, and then they just disappear. Why don't you test out your model in a middle-income neighborhood church or even in a church in an affluent neighborhood? See if you can prove that people who can afford to pay for any kind of medical care they need will choose a physician committed to wholistic and humanistic approaches. Up until now, all you have proven is that poor people who have no other place to go are willing to come into

a church for health care because it's free and available."
Others went on to say that we could always move back into the
poor neighborhoods after we had started one in an upper-
income neighborhood, but it would be difficult to go from a
poor neighborhood to an upper-income neighborhood.

So our second center was started under the sponsorship of
the W. K. Kellogg Foundation and the University of Illinois
Medical School in Chicago, Department of Preventive Medicine and Community Health. We chose Hinsdale, Illinois, a
western suburb of Chicago, and a Congregational church
with over two thousand active members.

We found that disseminating our "great idea" to that
sophisticated population in a western suburb of Chicago,
with more doctors per capita than any other western suburb,
was a frustrating experience. The people could not understand why their neighborhood had been chosen for a health
center when there were no poor people there. It just didn't
make sense. By and large, they were satisfied with the medical care they were receiving from their private physicians.
Most of them had three or four specialists with whom they
had a close working relationship. They were not about to turn
to us for medical care.

It took a year and a half for the general public in the surrounding suburban communities to grasp the concept, and
for a few to come as patients. However, before the general
population began to come, three distinct professional groups
began to show interest. First, after nurses of the area began
talking about it at their regular meetings, a trickle of nurses
who had been searching for a more humanistic approach to
health care began coming as patients. The second group was
social workers, whose enthusiasm for the concept spread even
beyond our own county so that we had social workers coming
from long distances. The third group was schoolteachers.
With their endorsement of the concept, new families moving
into the community inquiring about doctors were steered by
teachers in our direction.

During the entire first year and a half, we gave many
talks to service organizations, churches and so on, describing

the concept over and over again. Although there was always enthusiastic reception of the overall philosophy, there was also real skepticism as to "whether it could possibly be first-class medical care if it's done in a church." Somehow, most people had the idea that a doctor's office had to have all kinds of technical equipment which, of course, we did not. They equated good medicine with technology. About that time we saw fit to buy more stainless-steel equipment, which gave a certain feeling of satisfaction to many of our patients. We now began to look like a regular doctor's office.

We purposely tried to avoid any kind of newspaper publicity, but it inevitably came, and with it a large number of patients from a fifty-mile radius of Chicago. Most of those patients were "doctor hoppers" who soon discovered that our counseling approach could ferret out their unwillingness to change their lifestyle and their general attitude of "enjoying poor health." Not until about the third year did we begin to build a substantial clientele of patients from the immediate area who trusted us as a permanent part of the professional community.

It could be said that our suburban audience was more difficult to convince of the validity of our approach than was the low-income clientele in Springfield, Ohio. The suburban people, even though they responded enthusiastically to every presentation given to them, always thought of us as something good for someone else whom they knew. They were not ready to see themselves as needing an approach that took a look at their whole lifestyle as possibly contributing to illness. As we began offering a number of seminars and workshops for neighborhood people held in churches of many different denominations, it was as if they were saying, "Even though we are enthusiastic about your model, it's going to take us a few years to realize that we, too, need it. Also, we have doctors who are close friends, and we think that if we were to show too much interest in you for our own physical care, we would lose the right to go to them as specialists when we really need them."

That leads us to the most difficult group to disseminate

this concept to, namely, the physicians of the community. We sensed that some were so threatened by what we were proposing that it would not be wise for us to go into much detail about what we proposed to do. Another way to put it is to say that it was a good thing we didn't know exactly where we were going, because physicians were upset when we told them we were testing out a model of prevention and early detection of illness. In the early stages of 1973, if we had been able to say we were going into competition with them, we feel certain they would have found ways to stop us from continuing the project.

We felt it necessary to inform all 250 physicians in our area about our project, however, so we sent the following letter to them which described all that we were planning to do at that time. The fact that each center grew to look more and more like a family practice doctor's office, with additional components of counseling and continuing education for patients, was not all that clear in our minds in 1973.

Dear Doctor,

We want you to know about the Wholistic Health Center soon to open on Wednesday afternoons in Community Presbyterian Church, Clarendon Hills, and on Wednesday evenings at the Union Church of Hinsdale.

This is an action-research project of the Department of Preventive Medicine and Community Health of the Abraham Lincoln School of Medicine of the University of Illinois. It has been "approved in principle" by the DuPage County Medical Society and will be related to the Department of Health Education of the Hinsdale Sanitarium and Hospital.

The Wholistic Health Center will deal especially with one of the chief problems of health care—the approach of the patient to a doctor at the early signs of illness, instead of waiting until the illness is advanced.

The Wholistic Health Center will test new ways of encouraging people to get health care earlier in the course of illness. The Center will establish programs of health education and screening similar to those which the Hinsdale

Sanitarium has had for many years to detect heart disease.

We anticipate that the Center will attract a number of people who could be called the "worried well." The W.H.C. will have nurses and physicians available to determine which patients really need to be referred to direct medical care. The W.H.C. will also have trained counselors available to talk with those patients who mostly need someone with time to talk with them. Other patients will have the opportunity to participate in group discussions and seminars dealing with their particular kinds of complaints.

Physicians are invited to visit the Center and learn of its program. It may be that you will have patients who might respond well to our counseling and/or group health education program.

Of the 250 doctors who received that letter, only one called to say he felt it was an unnecessary project because doctors were practicing wholistic medicine anyway; he didn't appreciate the slur on present medical practice. We made a personal visit to his office and explained more in detail what our counseling procedures were like and how the educational courses were arranged. He agreed that he was not doing that much counseling or educating. He and a number of other doctors now send us patients with human problems.

Beyond the local level of physicians, we went to the county medical society and received their approval, which said that "we approve in principle" this project. Our relation to the national AMA had always been good inasmuch as I served on their Committee of Medicine and Religion for a ten-year period. That committee had approved the concept.

What We Have Learned
From the suburban Hinsdale experience, we feel that we learned the following things about disseminating wholistic health centers:

1. We felt that we had an idea whose time had not quite come but was in the process of becoming. Therefore we felt it essential that we give most of our attention to educating the community about the latest developments in psycho-

somatic medicine and wholistic insights.

2. The audience we were trying to reach were well-educated, suburban citizens who were beginning to read things having to do with changes in health care and the accent on a humanistic philosophy. Knowing that any new idea takes anywhere from ten to twenty years to come into full bloom, we were fortunate to have foundation help during the formative years when people were responding to the concept with mild enthusiasm but were not quite ready to invest their own money or their own lives in this kind of medical care.

3. I am convinced that if we had not had enthusiastic response from every neighborhood audience we addressed, we would not have attempted to start centers which require so much support and start-up funds. Actually, the only groups that were not enthusiastic were physicians. A few physicians in family practice and in departments of preventive medicine and primary care in medical schools have been quite encouraging.

4. Our progress in dissemination was assisted by the prominence of articles appearing in popular magazines, newspapers and even medical journals on the subject of stress and its contribution to illness.

5. My own work in the area of grief and loss convinced me that at least one-third of all patients seen by primary-care physicians have illnesses related to loss and grief. I assumed that, as popular emphasis on grief, death and dying helped people understand their relationship to illness, more physicians' offices would be needed where patients in the grief syndrome could be treated. The fact that a large number of clergy are well trained in that area led me to believe that we would be a much needed commodity.

6. We believe that our sense of timing was pretty much on target and that, although we preceded the public interest in wholism by three to five years, our present eight years of experience will stand us in good stead as we attempt to start several more wholistic health centers.

7. We were, in a sense, fortunate to be engaged in this project at a time of growing dissatisfaction with impersonal,

technologically oriented medical care by physicians. The fact that physicians were seeing patients for such brief times and charging such high rates also created a desire to find another pattern of health care.

8. In other words, the *kairos* was right. Any project that is too far ahead of its time will simply have to wait until people are ready for it. Recalling the old adage that "a king is king only as long as the people want him to be king," we operated under the assumption that people were tired of the scientific type of doctor as king and were in the process of unseating him as they sought a blend of science and humanism, however that might be arranged. Of course, that is exactly what we stress—that a medical doctor's office has to be a blend of both good, scientific medicine and warm, understanding humanism. We would not have been successful had we started such a program in 1960 because the population would not have been ready for it. Timing is essential to the dissemination of any new idea or, as with us, of an old idea in new dress.

Our second Chicago wholistic health center was started in Woodridge, a middle-income suburb with many young families, lots of mobility and instability, and no doctors. As a result, that center got off the ground much more quickly than the Hinsdale center and had the advantage of the good publicity which nearby Hinsdale now enjoyed. For Woodridge we did attempt some direct-mail publicity based on the newly approved right of doctors to advertise. We also found it helpful to have a health fair which attracted over six hundred people to the church. There, some twenty-five booths representing allied health programs in the Chicago area put the wholistic health center in the proper context of health institutions. In addition, morning coffees were held in many homes for women of the community. All these efforts helped to disseminate the work of the center.

It should be said that it was easier to explain the project in 1975 than in 1973 because two years had given many more people an introduction to wholistic medicine through articles in the press.

In 1976 we opened a center in rural Mendota, Illinois,

seventy miles west of Chicago. Among rural people we are finding it very difficult to disseminate the philosophy or to stir up much enthusiasm for the wholistic approach. Rural people are not accustomed to continuing education courses except on farm subjects, and they seem to have a kind of privateness about their physical ills. We are not at all sure how to deal with that problem and are about to call in some rural experts to help us in the marketing of our program.

We have no difficulty getting patients to come to the church-based center in Mendota, but that is because the physician in charge previously had her practice in the same town and simply moved her office into the church. Yet the counseling and the education courses are lagging in interest.

Our fourth center is in a low-income black neighborhood of inner-city Chicago where we are utilizing a former convent building for the center and including legal services as well as handicraft workshops for neighborhood people. Here we face quite a different problem in dissemination. The population is new to the community. They have moved in within the last few years and few of them have put down roots. There are no churches to speak of which have a regular congregation.

We have developed few handles with which to get hold of the problem of dissemination. But we have a core group of people as our center staff, representing a radical kind of congregation which chooses not to have a church building and rents a union hall for its services of worship. These people, who are also very committed to the neighborhood, have bought two apartment buildings, where they live. We have a group of some ten adults who are fully committed to health care. Two of the three physicians related to the center work half-time in emergency rooms; the other is assistant director of the family-practice residency program at Cook County Hospital. In that way, they can give up to fifty per cent of their time to the center as it grows, giving us a total of some sixty hours of professional medical services.

A fifth center in Oak Lawn, a southside suburb of Chicago, is related to a large hospital (Christ Hospital) of some eight hundred beds. There we are doing our disseminating of the project in conjunction with the public relations department of the local hospital, since the center will be operated by the hospital and its family-practice residency program.

Mobilizing Denominational Bodies

Perhaps the first thing that must be said is that there is a readiness on the part of people throughout the United States to listen to talks and lectures about wholism and humanizing health care. I have personally been disseminating information on wholistic concepts since the middle 1940s, when, as a hospital chaplain, I began speaking to lay and professional groups on behalf of the American Protestant Hospital Chaplains Association.

In the early '40s hospital boards of directors gradually realized that, although their hospitals often contained the name of a religious denomination, they were doing nothing about the spiritual dimension of illness. During those years, a few young chaplains (there were only a dozen in the entire country) formed what is now called the College of Hospital Chaplains. Within ten years it grew to over five hundred members. We see that growth as a quiet indication that people were saying something was missing in medical care and were beginning to identify it as the spiritual or humanistic ingredient.

So we are back again to the idea that to disseminate any new idea it is necessary that the people, or at least a certain percentage of the people, have a growing interest in that particular area of concern. If no one is interested or sensitive to an idea, dissemination of that idea will be difficult, perhaps impossible.

As I think about the national picture, however, I realize that large church bodies—denominations like Methodist, Presbyterian, Lutheran and others—have not developed an interest in health care to any great extent. As a matter of fact, even now denominational church bodies as such have not yet acknowledged any particular responsibility for health care, even though within their denomination scores or even hundreds of hospitals may bear their names.

To be sure, individuals within each denomination are raising the right kinds of questions concerning the responsibility of churches to participate in health care, but their voices are not yet heard by people in national staff positions. Other matters clamor for attention, and the staffs of the national churches have not yet seen health care as sufficiently important to their concerns to do anything significant about it. They are moving in that direction, however, without realizing it. As they show increasing interest in problems of the elderly, they indirectly get involved in long-term medical and custodial care of elderly people. The next step will be for them gradually to become aware of health care for the rest of the population as well.

I am living very close to the problem of how to disseminate wholistic health concepts to national church bodies, although I have been rebuffed up until now. I am convinced that lay people within the church are responding to our model clinics with such enthusiasm that they will eventually convey this concern to their leaders at the state and the national level. I have not yet figured out which buttons to push to make something happen sooner than it will happen by itself. I might consider organizing the "Associates of Wholistic Health Centers," inviting members to write or visit their key denominational church leaders and simply put pressure upon them to consider these ideas at a future annual meeting of their denomination.

Church bodies often operate on the basis of memorials or petitions initiated by smaller areas of their constituency. Since they are required to respond to them with some kind of answer, the following kinds of memorials might be developed.

A MEMORIAL TO_____SYNOD IN ASSEMBLY 1980: Regarding the need for the church at large to consider its role in reacting to the depersonalization of medical care by encouraging communication between religion and medicine.

WHEREAS the United States Government is, at this time, debating the national health insurance concept with a view to making equal care available to all people in America with total costs assumed by all of the people jointly; and

WHEREAS it has been noted that only three cents of the health dollar is now spent on preventive health care, and ninety-seven cents is spent on taking care of people after they get sick; and

WHEREAS the church has long been ministering to people of all types and conditions and has shown great effectiveness in fields akin to preventive medicine by providing opportunities for its members and others to find strength and hope through worship, fellowship, prayer and meditation; and

WHEREAS secular and even cultic answers to health problems are becoming tremendously popular with a population searching for ways to cope with the stresses and strains of life; and

WHEREAS half of the medical schools in America have within the last few years added faculty in medical ethics, indicating a growing interest in the moral and spiritual dimensions of illness; and

WHEREAS a new specialty in medicine called Family Practice Physicians has come into being during the past ten years to give new emphasis to a wholistic approach to health care which includes relating family, job and social and human concerns in the diagnostic process; and

WHEREAS suddenly a Society for Health and Human Values has grown from a dozen members to 2,000 members representing people in medical education and health care; and

WHEREAS over 50,000 clergy have received three months to two years of specialized clinical pastoral education in hospital and institutional settings preparing them to relate to the health care field;

WE NOW PROPOSE that our denomination take seriously its responsibilities to participate in the exciting new advances taking place in health-care policies and practices by employing a full-time "Secretary of Health" who will represent the church in the scores of seminars and study groups now being held throughout the world to make certain that the experience of the church through the ages is not lost as the health sciences seek to understand the human causes of illness and the ways in which we may cope with these causes.

We hope that when such a memorial is voted on in a local synod or state meeting, it will then move on up to the national convention as one or more synods decide to endorse it. When it reaches the national level, it is entirely possible that such a Secretary of Health will find himself or herself in conversation with key people in medical education, nursing education, hospital management and national health plans including Blue Cross. That should occur in a few years. If, at that time, we have perhaps twenty or thirty wholistic health centers as models for those in positions of leadership to study, the next steps will be relatively easy. Most national denominations, if they become convinced that a need is great enough, can automatically put one or more million dollars aside for that purpose. With that kind of money and with sufficient expertise built up by that time, it is our hope that wholistic health centers will provide a visible alternative style of primary health care. Physicians coming out of medical school will have another choice for location and style of practice which will be recognized as high-quality medical care.

Working with Other Groups
Our experience has been that many physicians who would like to relate to our wholistic approach feel that it is still too "far out." They think they would lose stature with their colleagues in medical practice if they were to join such a radical movement. As the radicalness of it disappears and it is seen as related to the two major institutions of our land, medicine and the church, it will not seem such a great risk to enter this kind of practice. Risk-taking is not as prevalent among doctors as some might imagine. Our experience has been that only about one per cent of doctors in America are willing to break with tradition to test out a new style of practice not approved by their colleagues. However, one per cent of

375,000 is 3,750 physicians who, if they heard about this concept, might be willing to test it out. If we have over 3,000 doctors who are open to this kind of idea, that is probably all we will need to make our point by about 1985. I would be gratified if, by 1985, there were 3,000 such centers in America. I am aware that it will take the approval of the AMA, the large denominations of churches, and the American Hospital Association to give it the impetus to happen.

I feel it is important to do new things within the context of the establishment. We have purposely taken no steps forward without consulting people in the AMA, in medical education and in the churches (including bishops) concerning what we intend to do. We have tried to maintain their respect and believe that we have succeeded. An article in the *AMA News* in June 1978 by president-elect Tom E. Nesbitt, M.D., said, "In my opinion, holistic health care with its counseling and educational functions can be a useful adjunctive component of our total health system."

We felt it would be wrong to stand on the outside and shout epithets at our elders in the establishment. It would not have been effective. We think our dreams are more certain of success when each step along the way is approved by people in positions of trust in the establishment.

To be sure, we have had to look hard. We long to find key people in various establishment positions who are willing to listen to what we have to say and then to encourage us. Such people make up perhaps only one to ten per cent of the leadership, yet we have been successful in finding these few who are in good repute in their particular groups. As they have spoken quietly but clearly about their approval of what we are doing, the sting has been taken out of our radical image. We have had less resistance from other establishment leaders because they know that we have been approved by some of their colleagues.

We regret that our image has been tarnished somewhat by newspaper writers lumping us together with other "holistic" people who espouse more radical concepts. Although we believe in much of their basic philosophy, our method of practice is more traditional. We have found it necessary to stress our traditional side so that we attract a cross-section of people. We must meet them first where they feel comfortable and then introduce them to methods of treatment that go beyond the physical dimension.

The one denomination in Christendom that I feel is now "ripe unto harvest" for consideration of the wholistic concept is the Roman Catholic Church. I sense this because of a sudden expression of interest by Catholic sisters who have long been related to hospitals. Their hospitals are now going through difficult times as they have lost sisters and have had to conduct their hospitals very much like secular institutions. Leadership among nuns has been meeting with some regularity to discuss the potential for increasing the spiritual dimension of health care even though they have a lack of religious personnel. During 1978, in several workshops with hospital-based Catholic nuns, I was excited by the unusual response they gave to our wholistic health-care concepts. I feel that it is only a matter of a year or two before we will see them begin to implement some experimental models in some of their many hospitals.

Another group whose readiness I believe is evident on all sides is the nursing professions. Some of them have been talking about wholistic approaches for at least two decades and their textbooks and journals are filled with recommendations of how to humanize health care. I find nurses to be the most enthusiastic audiences I have occasion to speak to. However, at the moment, in the health field the nursing profession has not been able to attain many important medical leadership roles. They have not been in a position to make policy decisions concerning how the health-care system should incorporate radically new modalities of health care. I see some gifted nurses relating to individual programs and exerting effective leadership, but the power of nurses is at a minimum in high-level policy decisions. That is regrettable.

It would be well for the dissemination of the wholistic idea if we could get to the boards of directors of hospitals through the good graces of the American Hospital Association. We have a great challenge to attempt to reach the administrators of hospitals who are now faced with poor public relations in the communities which they serve. People believe that hospitals are not interested in keeping people well but have a concern for them only when they are sick enough to fill a bed and pay a stiff fee for the use of that bed. Hospitals need to develop an image of concern for prevention and keeping people out of hospitals. If it is true that hospitals will be kept from adding the usual number of beds over the next several years and that they will be required to come up with new ways to serve their communities, that may produce an interest in preventive kinds of service to which hospitals can give support.

At the present time we are talking to half a dozen hospitals that have shown interest in the wholistic health center concept. Three of them are going ahead with model centers which will then be described to the hospital world through articles in hospital journals. I see this as an excellent way to get such centers underwritten for the costs of the start-up years, before becoming self-supporting from the third year on.

I also see a potential for relating all wholistic health centers to family-practice residency programs, which are in need of satellite locations to which residents can go to see different styles of health care and to participate in those new modes. Family-practice residency programs, which are limited to a hospital setting, are not giving their residents sufficiently broad experiences to equip them to be known as family physicians in neighborhood settings. Our intention is to continue to relate to the organization of teachers of family practice and also to locate new centers in close proximity to family-practice residency programs so that they will become visible and available to residents as one of their electives.

Medical schools generally are disinterested in wholistic medicine. Some centers should be located near medical schools for that reason, although we have less hope of interesting academically oriented faculty people in what we are doing. Yet we feel it a part of wisdom to do everything within our power to set up centers near medical schools so that their

visibility can shame the faculty into at least acknowledging
that there are other styles of health care with which they
should acquaint their students.

We need to take every possible channel of dissemination
seriously. As professionals and institutional board members
examine our wholistic models, they are invited to visit them.
They will continually hear about wholistic care from lay
people, who like our alternative style.

We sense that many medical professionals wish we would go
away. Yet we are confident of our future growth because we
believe intelligent lay people will eventually break through
the ultraconservative stance of physicians and force them to
take these new modes of health care seriously.

Chapter Nine

Terminal Care Models for Whole-Person Medicine

Balfour M. Mount

"Truly, I say to you, as you did it to one of the least of these my brethren, you did it to me" (Mt. 25:40).

Depersonalization as a Barrier to Care-Giving[1]
The explosion of medical information in recent times and the well-equipped hospitals of our affluent society have made possible an unprecedented standard of excellence in health care. Evidence suggests, however, that one cost of such progress has been a marked depersonalizing of our hospitals.

We in the health-care team often must become patients to appreciate the reality facing the recipient of health care. That underscores the fact that we are generally unaware of our deficiencies. The reasons for our lack of awareness, and indeed for our deficiencies, include: (1) the perceptual blinders we acquire through years of institutional conditioning during and after training; (2) our preoccupation with pathophysiology and the endemic pressures of medical future shock that keep us sharply focused toward investigating, diagnosing, prolonging life and curing; (3) the practice of placing a high value on technology and things cognitive, and of devaluing things affective, psychosocial and spiritual; and (4) our tendency to overestimate our sensitivity to the needs of others.

Does depersonalization occur in our hospitals? If so, why

does it occur? Does it influence the quality of patient care? What can we do about it?

In their landmark book *Sickness and Society,* Duff and Hollingshead[2] documented their exhaustive examination of the multidimensional factors other than physical disease that modify the care received by patients in hospitals. Their findings were sobering. More often than not, hospitalization was found to include a series of dehumanizing events. Patients were incorporated into the procedures of the institution so that eventually all sense of autonomy, identity and status as an individual was eliminated.

Depersonalization frequently starts in the admitting office where institutional power is expressed as the patient is made to wait. The process continues: patients are unable to wear their own clothes, leave the ward without notifying the persons in control, or take their own medications. Contact with the outside world is regulated and visiting hours are restricted.

The degree of depersonalization has been found to vary with the type of accommodation; it is most pronounced among the poorer socioeconomic groups in wards. The phrases "case load" and "clinical material" are symbolic of our tendency to perceive patients as objects and tools of learning rather than as persons who are the focal point of concern. The nurse-patient relationship is frequently technical, administrative and task-oriented rather than person-oriented, with nurses functioning primarily as administrators of the technology of medicine as ordered by physicians.

Duff and Hollingshead found that the extant physician-patient relationship (1) ruled out systematic appraisal of personal and family influences on symptoms, diagnosis and management; (2) was profoundly influenced by the social position of the patient; and (3) was rarely a simple one-to-one relation in the hospital but rather a varied association including private physicians, house staff and medical students. In only 11 per cent of patients was mental status perceived accurately by the physicians. Nursing personnel were even less perceptive in understanding the emotional status of the patients.[2]

Why do our hospitals spawn such depersonalization? The simplistic answer laypersons give, that physicians and nurses are interested only in their incomes and nonprofessional pursuits, and are "not what they used to be," seems inaccurate as we examine the motivations of the medical profession. Problems arise not through a lack of caring but because we set highly demanding occupational goals for ourselves— goals that are, for the most part, irrelevant to the "personhood" of the patient.

Another important factor in depersonalization is the power structure in the hospital. Patients have no power, whereas even in the formative training years health professionals are instilled with a role-related power that separates them from patients and from persons in other professions. The end result is an inequality that directly affects communication. Paul Tournier, the Swiss psychiatrist, noted, "When one dominates the other, there will no longer be a dialogue because one of the persons is eclipsed, his power of self-determination is paralyzed."[3]

Since this problem appears seriously to impair quality patient care, what corrective measures can be taken? Two basic factors must be recognized as a prelude to improving the situation: the uniqueness of the patient and the inherent limitations of our acute care institutions.

The central importance of recognizing the patient as a person has been emphasized by many physicians. Dunphy stated, "Frightened and uneasy, he needs more than anything to be recognized as a human being, not as a disease."[4] Peabody championed the same theme: "The treatment of disease may be entirely impersonal . . . but the care of the patient must be completely personal. . . . The secret of the care of the patient is in caring for the patient."[5]

But what does "caring for" a patient really mean? Mayeroff pointed out that to care for another person is to help that person grow toward self-realization.[6] Caring includes:

1. Profound respect for the "otherness" of other people, grounded in a sense of the individual's unique worth.

2. Helping others to care for themselves.

3. Meeting other people where they are rather than where we would like them to be.

4. Knowledge of other people's social context and needs.

5. Trust.

6. Humility and willingness to learn and receive from others.

7. A flexibility that enables change when mechanical application of the rules may not suffice.

8. An attitude toward care as not essentially a severe and strenuous demand placed on us in regard to others, but an opportunity to further our own development.[7]

What are the inherent limitations of our acute-care institutions in meeting these person-directed goals? The explosive increase in medical knowledge puts enormous demands on each of us as we try to maintain our expertise in pathophysiologic diagnosis and treatment. No one person can entirely meet the medical and personal needs of another. It follows that the medical system must incorporate person-oriented safeguards to caring.

Given these generalities, what specific recommendations can be made to assist us in our quest to humanize health care in hospitals? Although not comprehensive, the following list includes some methods of proven merit in reaching the goal:

1. Relax regulations concerning visiting, including visits by children.

2. Facilitate family-to-patient and patient-to-patient support by providing patient lounges and the possibility of privacy.

3. Employ a patient representative or ombudsman to identify the patient's needs and bring them to the attention of staff members.

4. When sizable ethnic minority groups form the patient body, acknowledge their customs concerning food and their need for privacy or, conversely, for continuing interaction in large family groups.

5. Improve recreational and diversional therapy programs.

Several changes can be made by hospital staff members in

their approach to patient care:

1. When entering a patient's room one should:

Address the patient by name.

Make eye contact with the patient before dealing with the IV bottle.

Always sit at the bedside no matter how short the visit, so that eye contact is on the same level. (A physician's visit will be remembered as being longer in duration and of greater meaning if the physician sits down.)

Acknowledge family members and other patients in a multiple-bed room.

Insure privacy during communication and examination.

Insure ample opportunity for private one-to-one communication with the patient. The presence of colleagues divides attention and invites division in how one relates to the patient.

Make an active effort to forget your professional role at some point during a visit. Do not be afraid to express personal feelings, but remember Shneidman's admonition: "A bed pan thrown at you should be interpreted, not reacted to."[8]

Be aware that approximately 70-90 per cent of communication by both patients and staff is nonverbal.

Honor the patient's need for privacy and independence, but remember that, for most patients, touching conveys an interest in the person and is reassuring.

2. Remember that adults, however sick, are not children and should not be patronized.

3. Increase emphasis on psychosocial and spiritual issues related to the patient and key family members by assessing these areas, in addition to medical concerns, at the time of admission, establishing distinct goals and drawing up intervention plans.

4. Utilize goal-oriented team conferences.

5. Establish the use of family conferences and invite relatives, nursing staff, physicians and other relevant team members.

6. Increase the use of social workers to define social goals

and to facilitate communication.

7. Include the chaplain in the ward management team.

8. Use volunteers as an integral and supportive part of the ward team.

9. Recognize the family's and patient's need for prompt information.

10. Organize multidisciplinary counseling teams to assist in high-risk situations, such as when patients are undergoing major surgery or abortion, when they are in the intensive-care unit or the emergency department or when they need terminal care.

11. Keep your sense of humor.

Caring for the Terminally Ill[9]

Two-thirds of the patients diagnosed as having cancer each year die of their malignancies.[10] Further, approximately 70 per cent of North Americans die in institutions.[11] In spite of these facts little effort has gone into sharpening our skills in treating patients with incurable disease. Indeed, evidence is increasing that such patients and their families experience a wide variety of critical problems that usually go unrecognized by those responsible for their care. The terminally ill patient, instead of receiving sympathetic understanding and expertise in meeting his medical and emotional needs, may encounter uncontrolled physical symptoms, isolation and particular depersonalization.[2 12 13 14]

Hinton has commented: "we emerge deserving of little credit; we who are capable of ignoring the conditions which make muted people suffer. The dissatisfied dead cannot noise abroad the negligence they have experienced."[15]

The Palliative Care Service at the Royal Victoria Hospital in Montreal was opened in January 1975. It has demonstrated that the needs of the terminally ill and their families can be met within the general hospital setting with a service that includes:

a trained multidisciplinary team;

a hospital ward, home visiting team and consultation service;

emphasis on specialized nursing care and the treatment of pain;

concern for patients' psychological, emotional and spiritual needs;

treatment and care of the patient and the family as a unit;

continuation of staff involvement with the family during bereavement.

Although this communication reflects Palliative Care Service experience with patients having advanced malignant disease, many of the observations may be relevant in other clinical settings.

Defining Appropriate Therapy

The current tendency to equate excellence of medical care with aggressive investigation and therapy is an outcome of the recent rapid expansion of medical knowledge. The result is a generation of physicians conditioned to see their role exclusively as "employed by the patient to fight for his life."[16] Failure to recognize that further investigation and active treatment may be inappropriate in the presence of advanced disease has frequently resulted in unnecessary suffering. We have often failed to recognize that the capacity to act does not, in itself, justify an action.

Three therapeutic goals are acceptable in the treatment of malignant disease: to cure, to prolong life, and to improve the quality of the remaining life. When therapy to prolong life is appropriate, unproven therapeutic modalities are justifiable only with informed consent as part of carefully designed and supervised clinical trials. Accepted forms of treatment may be justified only after a consideration of attendant morbidity, probability of response and mean duration of response, in consultation with the patient and family.

When enhanced quality of life becomes the only appropriate goal, further investigations should be carried out only if they lead to improved symptom control. Investigations for research purposes are justifiable in such a setting only when informed consent has been obtained from the patient.

The decision that therapy should be restricted to palliative care is made more easily if the physician's perception of his or her mandate embraces the broader concept of alleviating suffering rather than simply "fighting for life." The treater's need to treat, and the family's need to have treatment continued are unacceptable rationales for further therapy.

A decision that further "active therapy" is inappropriate should be associated not with a pessimistic attitude that "nothing more can be done," but with a positive statement that although therapy can no longer be expected to make an impact on the disease process, much can be done to control symptoms and assist the patient in living as fully and as comfortably as possible. It may be helpful to remind both patient and family that many medical problems, such as diabetes, arteriosclerotic vascular disease and multiple sclerosis cannot be cured, but that patients can lead a worthwhile life within the situation in the face of decreasing resources. The patient and family are left with the concept of an appropriate shifting in therapeutic goals by a physician who remains interested and actively engaged. The statement "nothing more can be done" reflects a tragic ignorance of the multidimensional needs of such patients and their families and the creative therapeutic responses to their needs that are now possible.

Nature of the Need

The traditional preoccupation of our health-care system with pathophysiology alone is especially inadequate in the arena of advanced disease. Although the medical needs may be undeniably complex and will be of great concern, added to them are complicating factors of psychological stress for the patient and family, strained interpersonal relationships, frequent financial problems and the ever-present spiritual questions such patients face: "Why me? Why this suffering? Why is this allowed? Is this all there is?" Experience suggests that intervention must be directed at all levels—physical, psychological, metaphysical or spiritual, and social—if suffering is to be successfully alleviated.

For the Christian physician, the endemic paucity of concern for psychosocial and spiritual issues in North American health care is of particular concern. It is important for us to recognize, however, that our Christian faith does *not* necessarily bestow on us particular clarity of perception concerning the needs of the terminally ill. In at least one study physicians describing themselves as "committed Christians" demonstrated the same important lack of awareness of the needs and feelings of dying patients as did agnostic physicians.[17] It may be tempting for us to approach the patient with answers without taking the time to determine the true nature of the questions at hand.

The sobering reality is that terminally ill patients are likely to receive unacceptably inadequate physical care at our hands. That this is not good enough is suggested by James 2:15-17, "If a brother or sister is ill-clad and in lack of daily food, and one of you says to them, 'Go in peace, be warmed and filled,' without giving them the things needed for the body, what does it profit? So faith by itself, if it has no works, is dead." Our current documented inadequacies must be doubly disheartening as we hear Christ admonish us, "Truly, I say to you, as you did it not to one of the least of these, you did it not to me" (Mt. 25:45).

Chronic Pain

When the intractable pain of malignant disease is present, its treatment is the central focus in palliative care.

Nature of chronic pain.   It is important to recognize the significant difference between acute and chronic pain. Acute pain has a beginning and an end. It may be classified as mild, moderate or severe and has a "purpose" in that it draws attention to the offending member so that corrective therapy may be introduced. Chronic pain, however, can be characterized as a vicious circle with no set time limit. Fearful anticipation of its perpetuation leads to anxiety, depression and insomnia, which in turn accentuate the physical components of the pain.[18] Leshan suggests that meaninglessness, helplessness and hopelessness are characteristic of the unreal nightmare world in which the patient with chronic pain lives.[19] Pain forcefully reminds patients with advanced malignant disease of their prognosis, thus increasing their distress. Saunders has coined the term "total pain" to describe the multiple components of chronic pain—physical, psychological, spiritual and social.[20]

Aims of treatment. The goals of the therapist should be:

1. Identifying the etiology: Clarification of the cause is an essential first step in pain control since it may lead to specific therapy, such as focal irradiation for a bony metastasis, extraction of a carious tooth or bowel care for pain due to constipation.

2. Preventing pain: The aim is to anticipate and prevent pain rather than treat it. This requires regular administration of appropriate amounts of analgesic, at a dose titrated against the patient's current needs. There is no place for "prn" medication orders as the standard for treatment of chronic pain, since the resultant pattern of recurring pain produces unnecessary suffering and escalation in analgesic dose.

3. "Erasing" pain memory: As the anxious anticipation and memory of pain is lessened by successful pain prevention, the dose of analgesics required can frequently be decreased.

4. An unclouded sensorium: Many patients feel trapped between perpetual pain on the one hand and somnolence on the other. A pain-free state without sedation requires careful individual regulation of analgesic dose according to the patient's need.

5. A normal affect: The ability of a patient to relate to his environment will be enhanced if the agents used to control pain do not inappropriately elevate or depress mood.

6. Ease of administration: Oral administration of analgesics can allow a patient to retain a degree of independence and mobility that is impossible when analgesics are given parenterally. Cachexia may also make regular intramuscular injections difficult and painful.

Management of chronic pain. If the pain is localized, radiation therapy, nerve block or some form of ablative neurosurgical procedure may provide excellent control.

With moderate to severe chronic pain, only the narcotic analgesics provide adequate control. Milder analgesic should always be tried for less severe pain and may be helpful in combination with more potent drugs. A wide variety of agents is available: Catalano has provided a helpful review.[21]

In the past the use of narcotics for chronic pain has been widely considered "bad management." Recent studies have demonstrated, however, that all the above treatment goals may be achieved using oral narcotics, without danger of tolerance and attendant dose escalation. An oral narcotic mixture containing morphine, taken in conjunction with a phenothiazine, has provided excellent pain control in 75-80 per cent of patients with intractable cancer pain in general hospital accommodations and in 90 per cent of patients in the Palliative Care Unit.[22] The remainder, with very few exceptions, had excellent pain control with regularly given parenteral narcotics prescribed with a phenothiazine.

One standard formulation for an oral mixture is a variable amount of morphine, 10 mg of cocaine, 2.5 ml of flavoring syrup and a variable amount of chloroform water for a total of 20 ml per dose. The mixture is given regularly, every four hours around the clock in conjunction with a phenothiazine syrup, usually prochlorperazine starting at 5 mg per dose. In the presence of restlessness, chlorpromazine, starting at 10 mg per dose, may be used instead of prochlorperazine.

Lengthy anticipated patient survival is not a contraindication to narcotic use since, with careful dosage adjustment, the mixture can be used for periods extending to several years without dose escalation.

For most patients, pain relief can be obtained with 5-10 mg of morphine Q4h, while in small or elderly patients as little as 2.5 mg may be effective. A pain-free state can be achieved in most patients by giving sequential increments in the narcotic dose (Figure 9.1). The usual dosage range of morphine given in the mixture is 2.5 to 30 mg but doses of 120 mg have been used; the usual increment is 5-10 mg per dose.

For excruciating pain, an alternative method is to start with a relatively high narcotic dose, subsequently adjusting the dose in sequential decrements until analgesia without sedation is achieved. Since narcotics and the phenothiazines are

Figure 9.1[24]

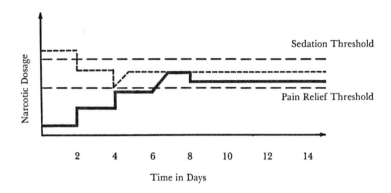

Alternative methods of dosage adjustment. Pain relief in the absence of sedation may be achieved with sequential increments in narcotic dose at intervals of 2 days (_____). In a few cases the severity of the pain will require an initially high dose, followed by sequential decrements until the pain reappears (. . . . . .). A slight increase in dose provides analgesia without sedation.

synergistic, the dose of only one variable—the narcotic or the phenothiazine—should be changed at a time. Even small dose alterations may lead to profound changes in analgesia and sedation. The physician's confident reassurance that pain can be controlled undoubtedly has a beneficial effect in promoting analgesia.

Dispensing the morphine mixture and the phenothiazine syrup separately allows greater flexibility while adjusting the doses. Once a continuous pain-free state is achieved, they may be combined in dispensing for greater ease of administration.

Careful observation of the patient's condition over a complete twenty-four-hour period may suggest augmentation of one or two specific doses at periods of peak activity.

If parenteral medication becomes necessary, the equivalent dose of morphine is roughly one-half the previous oral dose. Thus a patient whose pain has been controlled with 30 mg of morphine taken orally would require about 15 mg intramuscularly.[23][24]

Adverse effects.   Adverse effects are infrequent with this approach. Effects to be watched for include sedation, nausea and vomiting, constipation, respiratory depression, tolerance/dependence and extrapyramidal effects. The potentiation of the narcotic sedation effect by the phenothiazine has been referred to earlier. It is important to reassure both patient and family that the initial drowsiness associated with the introduction of narcotics is temporary, lasting only forty-eight to seventy-two hours. After the initial forty-eight hours, sustained sedation suggests that the narcotic dose is excessive. However, if the physician, fearful of narcotics, has delayed their introduction until the final days or weeks of life, the patient may well be more drowsy and less communicative when the pain is finally controlled. In advanced malignant disease there is often increased weakness, somnolence and occasionally confusion. The physician should explain to the family that such changes in mental status are not caused by medication but are secondary to advancing disease (hepatic or renal insufficiency, other metabolic problems, or intracranial metastases) in most instances.

Nausea and vomiting, a common side effect of narcotics, is countered by the routine use of phenothiazines. If a patient is vomiting before therapy is instituted, control should first be achieved with parenteral medication prior to switching to the oral route.

The combined effect of poor dietary intake, dehydration, inactivity and narcotic therapy almost invariably leads to constipation. It should be prevented by using a combination of a stool softener and a bowel stimulant such as Dioctyl sodium sulfosuccinate and Senna concentrate.

Clinically significant respiratory depression and tolerance, with associated dose escalation, are rarely encountered when the dose has been carefully titrated to the patient's need. Marks and Sachar have commented that "the excessive and unrealistic concern about the danger of addiction in the hospitalized medical patient is a significant and potent force for

undertreatment with narcotics."[25] It appears that undertreatment with analgesic medication may encourage craving and
psychological dependence. Our own experience confirms
that of Twycross that a change in dosage requirements her-
alds a change in disease status rather than tolerance.[22] [23]

Recent experience with the use of morphine in conjunction
with the phenothiazine, but without the other additives of the
mixture, suggests that this simplified approach may be equally effective in pain control.[26] Figure 9.2 gives details of the
oral narcotic mixture currently employed at our hospital.

Moreover, potent narcotics other than morphine, given at
appropriate intervals (allowing for their various half-lives),
can be used in similar treatment regimens against chronic
pain. Oral methadone, Levorphanol, oxycodone (also available in suppository form), anileridine, or hydromorphone
can be administered regularly with dosage titrated to the patient's need. Careful assessment of the patient's psychological
status may lead to judicious use of tricyclic antidepressants
and the benzodiazepines. Anti-inflammatory agents, such as
phenylbutazone (particularly with bone pain), corticosteroids
and hypnotics, may all be useful adjuncts in attacking the
vicious circle of chronic pain. The presence of a positive
supportive environment is seen as a further factor in decreasing pain and assisting in its control.[18] [22]

Control of Physical Symptoms Other Than Pain

The shifting symptom complexes and diminishing resources
of the terminally ill require regular and frequent reassess-
ment for symptom control. Such a practice will pay rich divi-
dends in the avoidance of potentially serious problems and
unnecessary hospitalization. The implied message that the
physician has a continuing interest in the patient's welfare
is a reassuring factor of major importance to both patient
and family. Figure 9.3 outlines methods commonly employed
in the control of physical symptoms other than pain.

Of particular note is the experience of Saunders in medical
management of malignant bowel obstruction.[24] She has observed that such obstruction is usually temporary and that

Figure 9.2[26] Effects of Brompton mixture and oral morphine solution on pain, confusion, nausea and drowsiness

Crossover Design	Morphine in mixture Mean Score (mg)	Pain Intensity Mean Score	Confusion Mean Score	Nausea Mean Score	Drowsiness Mean Score
Group I (N = 20)					
Brompton mixture	26.8	1.8	0.1	0.8	1.0
Morphine solution	24.5	1.7	0.1	0.3	1.1
P value	.19	.75	1.0	.06	.70
Group II (N = 7)					
Brompton mixture	18.0	1.6	0.1	0	0.7
Morphine solution	21.4	1.6	0.1	0	1.4
P value	.67	.93	1.0	1.0	.05
Independent Sample Design					
Brompton mixture (N = 11)	21.4	1.9	0.2	0.5	1.2
Morphine solution (N = 6)	15.8	1.9	0.2	0.7	1.3
P value	.39	.92	.94	.65	.77

Figure 9.3[9]

Symptom	Comment	Therapy
Anorexia	very common important effect on general status and morale reassure patient and com- pulsive family that large intake unnecessary	glucocorticosteroids, (prednisone 5 mg tid) small food helpings on small plates patient's preferred foods control subliminal nausea
Nausea and Vomiting	variety of causes including bowel obstruction, tumor bleeding, metabolic upset, psychological, drugs with reassurance, vomiting is well tolerated in the absence of nausea	if oral narcotic related, switch narcotics; try suppository (e.g. oxycodone) use with phenothiazine (prior to parenteral); once nausea controlled try oral route again. phenothiazines (in order of ascending seda- tive effect) a) prochlorperazine 5-10 mg b) promazine 25 mg c) chlorpromazine 10-25 mg (PO, IM, PR) for further control may add to the pheno- thiazine one or both of the following: a) cyclizine 50 mg PO or IM bid b) metoclopramide 10 mg PO or IM 1 hour ac tid small feeds of favorite foods see text re: bowel obstruction
Dysphagia	varies from mild and occasional to pronounced and present with all oral intake	eliminate nonessential drugs use PO liquid drugs or suppositories crush tablets and mix with ice cream small liquid or soft feeds of favorite foods honey solutions and iced carbonated drinks local anesthetics (with care) scrupulous and frequent mouth care treat monilia with nystatin suspension or vaginal suppositories sucked orally

**Dry Mouth:
Thirst
Dehydration**
	N.B.—thirst = symptom
	(unpleasant)
	dehydration = metabolic
	state (can be
	asymptomatic)
	often drug related
	intravenous fluids and
	nasogastric tube
	generally not justifiable!
	dry mouth is common;
	watch for and treat
		mouthwash q2h. lip-salve or bland cream
		for lips
		remove encrustations with water soluble
		(catheter) lubricant followed by gauze swab
		wipeout
		eliminate causative drugs if possible
		give lemon candies, pineapple chunks,
		artificial saliva
		remove foreign objects from mouth
		treat—candidiasis (see monilia)
		   stomatitis due to chemotherapy
		    astringent mouthwash
		    topical anesthetic
		ice chips, favorite drink, water sips (by syringe
		or eyedropper if too weak to use straw)

Hiccoughs	irritating and exhausting	rebreathing air into paper bag chlorpromazine 25 mg PO or IM breath-holding
Dyspnea	often associated with anxiety common causes are pleural effusion and lymphan-	calm, quiet reassurance with frequent observation, open window, fan positioning in bed or reclining chair

	gitic tumor spread less common are bronchial obstructions, massive ascites or abdominal tumor	mouth care oxygen? (often of little help) thoracentesis + instillation of chemothera- peutic agents for malignant pleural effusion bronchodilators (P.R.N., bronchospasm) oxytriphylline (choledyl) 40 mg qid salbutamol (Ventolin) by inhaler aminophyllin suppositories 1-2 prn also IV, PO. glucocorticosteroids prednisone 10-15 mg tid tapering to 5 mg tid antibiotics for symptomatic control in presence of purulent sputum trimethoprim + sulphamethoxazole ampicillin chloramphenical narcotics narcotic oral mixture (see text re: pain) or parenteral narcotic with phenothiazine or diazepam or alone
Terminal Airway Secretions ("Death Rattle")	often disturbing for families, rarely for patients themselves	hyoscine 0.4-0.6 mg prn
Cough	tiring, particularly at night N.B., if patient already on significant dose of nar- cotic for pain, do not add narcotic (e.g., codeine) for cough	linctus codeine or other narcotic, at night particularly bronchodilators, antibiotics, physiotherapy, hydration, where appropriate expectorants of questionable benefit
Anxiety	common factor in escalating pain and analgesic requirements	discussion and support are the primary therapies diazepam 2-5 mg tid PO: 10 mg IM or IV in acute panic states promazine 25 mg tid PO chlorpormazine 10-25 mg tid PO
Depression	not all depression requires medication: anticipatory grief is an integral com- ponent of the normal response to life-threaten- ing illness	attention to physical and mental distress tricyclic antidepressants imipramine 25-100 mg amitriptyline 25-100 mg given HS starting at low dose and increasing
Confusion Restlessness	variety of etiologic factors requiring careful evaluation often correctable by non- pharmacological means	reality reinforcement including calendars, clocks, orientation tours, repeated identification of familiar objects and events, photographs, social interaction haloperidol 1-4 mg q4-6h may be useful elevated intracranial pressure: dexametha- sone trial 4 mg tid if agitated, chlorpromazine 10-25 mg (mild) or 25-50 mg (severe), IM
Insomnia	adequate sleep important with diminished reserves	attention to physical and mental distress rituals: warm water bottle, hot drink, "well- timed bedpan," change of position, quiet,

		shaded lights, alcohol nonbarbiturate hypnotics chlorpromazine 25-50 mg tricyclic antidepressants or narcotic analgesics, if already in use but not simply as hypnotics waken for regular 4 hourly narcotic dose if analgesia inadequate throughout night
Urinary Symptoms Incontinence		take to bathroom frequently leave urine bottle close by condom for nocturnal incontinence catheter for constant incontinence or for retention, with maintenance urinary antiseptic treat symptomatic infections only
Constipation	debilitation, dehydration, drugs, immobility all contribute common prevent rather than treat	increased fluid and bulk (bran) when tolerated glycerine suppositories, disposable phosphate enema stool softener (e.g., Na dioctyl sulfosuccinate) plus peristaltic agent (e.g., senna) digital disimpaction
Diarrhea	rule out constipation with overflow	codeine 15-60 mg tid or Lomotil^R 2 qid bismuth subgallate 500 mg tid may be useful for unpleasant colostomy or fistula odors
Fungating Growths	need not be offensive	scrupulous cleanliness frequent dressing change wash with dilute dakins or peroxide solutions malodorous infections may respond to yoghurt applications rarely, systemic antibiotics for infection with associated foul discharge
Pruritis	common with obstructive jaundice; may be intolerable	rule out sensitivity to linen calamine lotion with phenol up to 1% hydrocortisone cream oral antihistamines
Decubitus Ulcers	common in older patients rare in young patients even if very cachectic and immobile	prevent with mobilization, physiotherapy, frequent position change, massage, reclining chairs camp air mattress on bed, half-filled with water, is an excellent, economic water bed if small and shallow, frequent cleansing with dakins if deep, 20% benzoyl peroxide-soaked pad to stimulate granulation, packed in wound under air-tight cellophane dressing: sur- rounding intact skin protected with vasoline or silicone cream (Barriere^R), U.V. light, physiotherapy

with the passage of time most will open up to allow passage of flatus and stool. Of further importance is her observation that vomiting is well tolerated in the absence of nausea. Malignant bowel obstruction may be managed with rigorous mouth care to control thirst, oral intake as desired, careful titration of medications to control nausea as per Figure 9.3, the use of softening laxatives such as Dioctyl sodium sulfosuccinate (Dioctyl Forte^R tabs) 1 or 2 tid, and reassurance to minimize the psychological trauma of vomiting. Diphenoxylate hydrochloride plus atropine (Lomotil^R) tabs 2 qid may be used to control painful colic. Frequency of vomiting will depend on the level of the bowel obstruction. In the great majority of cases malignant bowel obstruction resolves even if it has persisted for prolonged periods (up to twenty-six days in the author's experience). This approach provides patient comfort without resorting to colostomy, nasogastric suction or intravenous fluids.

When death is imminent, a standing order for hyoscine 0.4 to 0.6 mg, to be given SC, prn, is of great assistance in controlling the noisy respirations or "death rattle" so distressing to relatives, if not to the patient, during the final hours of life. Morphine and chlorpromazine given IM are useful in relieving distress stemming from a major crisis such as hemorrhage or massive pulmonary embolus. Their use in this setting, for the control of symptoms only, differs significantly from the prescribing of drugs with the intent of shortening life. If their use leads to an insignificant shortening of life, that is an accepted risk, taken in the interest of alleviating suffering. A clear understanding of the goals will alleviate anxiety on the part of nursing staff in such a situation.

Mental Distress in the Setting of Terminal Illness

The terminal patient is nearly always either consciously or unconsciously aware that death is close.[12][28] Kubler-Ross has suggested a series of mental adjustments which many go through in coming to terms with the fact that they have a serious or life-threatening disease. The series includes denial, anger, bargaining, depression and finally acceptance. Whatever the sequence in a given patient, one can usually find a subtle balance between a realistic acceptance on the one hand and simultaneous rejection on the other. In dying we are challenged to adapt, not to a single loss, but rather to a series of losses: job, mobility, strength, physical and mental capacity, plans for the future and, ultimately, existence itself.

The patient's family will go through a similar series of mental adjustments. An understanding of that process will assist the physician in accepting the anger of the patient or relative when it is redirected at him and in mediating more skillfully when anger is directed at a family member. Depression may call for a lengthy discussion and a listening ear rather than a consultation from a neurologist or psychiatrist, or the ordering of antidepressant medications.

Through understanding the dynamics of adjusting to death, physicians may realize more clearly the degree to which they share in the same series of mental adjustments as they face a patient's death. They may then recognize with greater clarity that avoidance of contact with the patient reflects their own despair. The physician's attitude toward his or her own death has been found to be an important variable in determining how they perceive a patient's needs: 84 per cent of Royal Victoria Hospital physicians who felt they would want to know their own prognosis if they were fatally ill thought their patients also desired direct communication of prognosis, while only 45 per cent of physicians not wanting to know their own prognosis thought their patients desired honesty of communication.[29] Our skill at "hearing" our patients will also depend on our recognition that they use not only plain language, but also figurative speech and nonverbal communication in expressing their fears and needs to us.[12]

Fears of the dying.   At least seven common fears are associated with dying. Fear of pain and mutilation is frequently encountered. A realistic appraisal of potential problems, and reassurance that they will be dealt with, will go a long way toward allaying relevant anxieties and will dispel many irrelevant concerns that are linked in the patient's mind to the fearful term "cancer." As noted above, the intractable pain of advanced malignant disease can generally be controlled using oral narcotics, leaving the patient alert and pain-free.

A second important fear is that of isolation. Patients with advanced disease are likely to encounter decreasing interest and fewer visits from a physician and members of the nursing staff if they are in the hospital, and from friends if they are at home. A recent study of eighty breast carcinoma patients revealed that their fear of isolation was greater than the fear of the disease itself, inadequate care and all other variables mentioned.[30] Reassurance from the physician that he or she will continue to supervise the patient's care with interest and concern and use of this opportunity to facilitate family discussions and expression of feeling are effective weapons in combating isolation.

A third fear is that of loss of control and of increasing dependence. This is particularly a problem for the previously self-reliant individual. It is important to recognize that the process of depersonalization, discussed earlier, may be particularly marked for such patients.

A fourth area of fear is for the future of the patient's loved ones. "What will happen to them after I die?" It is important for the patient to express such concerns and if possible to participate with the family in preparing for the future.

A further anxiety has been termed "reflected fear," the fear the patient sees in the eyes of others. This was commented on by a young cancer patient who stated, "I never knew what fear was until I saw it in the eyes of those caring for me."

Two other fears commonly seen in the terminally ill are fear of the unknown and fear that life has no meaning. The former tends to center around practical questions. "How will I die?" "Will I suffer?" The latter implies a consideration of major metaphysical issues. The perceptive physician has an opportunity to help patients express such questions and formulate their own answers.

For the Christian, whether the giver of care or the patient, the apostle Paul's words (Rom. 8:38-39) are a source of comfort in this setting, "For I am sure that neither death, nor life, nor angels, nor principalities, nor things present, nor things to come, nor powers, nor height, nor depth, nor anything else in all creation, will be able to separate us from the love of God in Christ Jesus our Lord." We are thus able to say with Isaiah, "In quietness and in trust shall be your strength" (Is. 30:15).

In rejoicing that our faith may be "more than sufficient" we will be wise to recognize that the psychological resources of even the most mature Christian will be modified by a variety of factors in addition to faith. Those factors have been listed by Parkes[31] (Figure 9.4). Even a "giant in the faith" like C. S. Lewis has faced an abyss of unexpected doubt and despair in the face of death. Following the death of his wife Lewis wrote: "In which sense is my faith a house of cards? Because the things I am believing are only a dream or because I only dream that I believe them?"[32]

Understanding that doubts may occur and that they are not so much a measure of the absence of faith as a natural extension of our human limitations of perspective will allow us to minister to each other more helpfully, until, as in C. S. Lewis's case, the dawn of new faith once again appears at the end of the darkness.

Cancer is frequently associated with serious threats to the patient's body image and concept of self. Problems requiring particular understanding and supportive discussion include:

Disfigurement due to radical surgery.

Alterations in body image particularly where sexual function is concerned.

Necessity of urinary or fecal diversion.

Loss of hair and other side effects of irradiation and chemotherapy.

Time must be taken to talk through the implications of each problem and the anxieties they produce.

Conspiracy of silence.   Uncertainty leads to anxiety. The reluctance of patient, family and physician to discuss frankly the reality facing them has been referred to as the "conspiracy of silence." A candid, honest, yet supportive approach will

Figure 9.4[33] Determinants of the Outcome of Bereavement[31]

Antecedent

Childhood experiences (especially losses of significant persons)

Later experiences (especially losses of significant persons)

Previous mental illness (especially depressive illness)

Life crises prior to the bereavement

Relationship with the deceased

        Kinship (spouse, child, parent, etc.)

        Strength of attachment

        Security of attachment

        Degree of reliance

        Intensity of ambivalence (love/hate)

Mode of death

        Timeliness

        Previous warnings

        Preparation for bereavement

        Need to hide feelings

Concurrent

Sex

Age

Personality

        Grief proneness

        Inhibition of feelings

Socioeconomic status (social class)

Nationality

Religion (faith and rituals)

Cultural and familial factors influencing expression of grief

Subsequent

Social support or isolation

Secondary stresses

Emergent life opportunities (options open)

produce less anxiety in the long run than well-intentioned dishonesty or a lack of communication. The conspiracy of silence hinders the patient's relationship with others. Further, it is a spreading process, with dishonesty about diagnosis and prognosis leading to the need for distortions in other matters.

Although there is need for supportive honesty in dealing with the terminally ill, the physician must not break down a patient's need for denial. The physician must also honor the need for "hope," without misunderstanding what the patient is hoping for. A plea for cure or a longer life, long after the patient realizes that these are no longer reasonable goals, may in fact be an expression of fear. For most terminally ill patients a desire for longer life gives way to other hopes: hope for an absence of pain, for skilled nursing care and for a family and physician who will stay at hand until the end.

The physiological explanation of "out of the body" experiences described by some individuals near death remains uncertain. Such experiences are often disturbing to the patient, who may feel they are losing touch with reality and thus tell no one of the event. On the other hand they may be deeply impressed by the experience, describing it in detail to relatives and friends, thus heightening their anxiety. The knowledge that such dramatic occurrences may be a part of an encounter with death for emotionally stable, objective and reliable individuals is reassuring to all concerned.

At the Time of Death

Most patients do not fear death itself but pain in dying. In reality, however, when death comes it is usually painless and peaceful for a patient dying of malignant disease. Mental and physical pain commonly recede during the last few days and almost always in the last hours. The reassurance that this is so may encourage a family to keep their loved one at home when their anxiety would otherwise necessitate hospitalization. The family will need particular support and guidance if the patient is to die at home. The assistance of a home-care nurse to supervise the administration of medications during the final days is invaluable. It is also important that the family be aware of the community resources available to them. A social worker may be of great assistance. Anxieties are lessened if the family has discussed funeral arrangements before the death.

It is often expected that the physician will come to the

bedside when the patient dies. Although this is not always possible, it should be a definite goal for the physician primarily involved in the case. He or she can make an important contribution toward resolution of the family's immediate problems and future "grief work," by being present at that critical point.

On the Palliative Care Unit a brief commemorative act on the part of the physician or nurse present at the time of death declares that something of significance has happened. A prepared memorial prayer has been useful in this regard. It tends to ease the tension of the moment and has invariably been meaningful regardless of the family's religious background.

Although the needs of the patient end with death, the family's needs continue. Normal and pathological grief reactions have been well described by Lindemann and Parkes.[33] [31] Our experience supports the observation, made by Parkes, that bereavement follow-up by a nurse or physician involved in the death makes an important difference to successful resolution of the family's grief.

Conclusion

The complex medical needs of terminal patients and the importance of psychological, spiritual and interpersonal considerations place special demands on physicians. They are required to be an internist skilled in the fine titration of medications against symptoms, a psychiatrist, a philosopher, a chaplain and a social worker. But the end of life is also a time of unparalleled potential for personal and interpersonal growth for patients and their families. Having assisted in the realization of that potential, the physician may share in the growing process.

Higher standards of care must be set if we are to write an end to unnecessary suffering of the terminally ill. The onus is on each of us to examine and improve standards of care in our own institutions.

Notes

[1] Balfour M. Mount, "Caring in Today's Health Care System," *Canadian Medical Association Journal,* 119 (1978), 303.

[2] R. S. Duff and A. B. Hollingshead, *Sickness and Society* (New York: Harper, 1968), p. 213.

[3] Paul Tournier, *The Meaning of Persons* (London: SCM Press, 1957), p. 137.

[4] J. E. Dunphy, "Annual Discourse—On Caring for the Patient with Cancer," *New England Journal of Medicine,* 295 (1976), 313.

[5] F. W. Peabody, "The Care of the Patient," *Journal of the American Medical Association,* 88 (1927), 877.

[6] M. Mayeroff, *On Caring* (New York: Harper & Row, 1971), p. 1.

[7] J. B. Nelson, *Human Medicine: Ethical Perspective on New Medical Issues* (Minneapolis, Minn.: Augsburg, 1973), p. 29.

[8] E. S. Shneidman, "Some Aspects of Psychotherapy With Dying Patients," paper presented at Psychological Care of the Dying Patient conference, San Francisco (2-3 June 1978).

[9] Balfour M. Mount, "Palliative Care of the Terminally Ill," *Annals of the Royal College of Physicians and Surgeons of Canada* (July 1978), p. 201.

[10] C. Holden, "Hospices: For the Dying, Relief from Pain and Fear," *Science,* 193 (1976), 389.

[11] Statistics Canada, *Vital Statistics,* Bulletin 3 (1973), p. 61.

[12] Elizabeth Kubler-Ross, *On Death and Dying* (New York: Macmillan, 1969).

[13] L. Lasagna, "Physicians' Behavior Toward the Dying Patient," in *The Dying Patient,* eds. O. G. Brim, H. E. Freeman, S. Levine et al. (New York: Russell Sage, 1970).

[14] Balfour M. Mount, "The Problem of Caring for the Dying in a General Hospital: The Palliative Care Unit as a Possible Solution," *Canadian Medical Association Journal,* 115 (1976), 119.

[15] J. Hinton, *Dying,* 2nd ed. (Harmondsworth, England: Penguin, 1972), p. 159.

[16] F. H. Epstein, "The Role of the Physician in the Prolongation of Life," in *Controversy in Internal Medicine,* eds. F. J. Ingelfinger, R. V. Ebert, M. Finland and A. S. Relman (Philadelphia: W. B. Saunders, 1974).

[17] Balfour M. Mount, "Christian and Agnostic Attitudes Toward Death," *Ontario Medical Review* (January 1974), p. 11.

[18] R. Melzack, "The Medical Approach to Management of Pain Caused by Cancer," in *The Puzzle of Pain* (Harmondsworth, England: Penguin, 1973).

[19] L. Leshan, "The World of the Patient in Severe Pain of Long Duration," *Journal of Chronic Diseases,* 17 (1964), 119.

[20] C. Saunders, *The Management of Terminal Illness* (London: Edward Arnold Publishers Ltd., 1978).

[21] R. B. Catalano, "The Medical Approach to Management of Pain Caused by Cancer," *Seminars in Oncology,* 2 (1975), 379.

[22] R. Melzack, J. G. Ofiesh and B. M. Mount, "The Brompton Mixture: Effects on Pain in Cancer Patients," *Canadian Medical Association Journal,* 115 (1976), 125.

[23] R. Twycross, "Clinical Experience with Diamorphine in Advanced

Malignant Disease," *International Journal of Clinical Pharmacology,* 9 (1974), 184.

[24]B. M. Mount, I. Ajemian and J. F. Scott, "The Use of the Brompton Mixture in Treating the Chronic Pain of Malignant Disease," *Canadian Medical Association Journal,* 115 (1976), 122.

[25]M. D. Marks and E. J. Sachar, "Undertreatment of Medical In-Patients With Narcotic Analgesics," *Annals of Internal Medicine,* 78 (1973), 173.

[26]R. Melzack, B. M. Mount and J. M. Gordon, "The Brompton Mixture Versus Oral Morphine: Effects on Pain," *Canadian Medical Association Journal,* 120 (1979), 435-38.

[27]C. Saunders, "The Nursing of Patients Dying of Cancer," *Nursing Times,* 72 (1976), 19.

[28]C. B. Bahnson, "Psychologic and Emotional Issues in Cancer: The Psychotherapeutic Care of the Cancer Patient," *Seminars in Oncology,* 2 (1975), 293.

[29]B. M. Mount, A. Jones and A. Patterson, "Death and Dying: Attitudes in a Teaching Hospital," *Urology,* 4 (1974), 741.

[30]B. Hoerni, F. Vedelago, C. Guillon and C. Lagarde, "Difficultes Socio-psychologiques pour le Diagnostic, l'Hospitalisation et le Traitement des Femmes Atteintes de Cancer du Sein," *Deuxiemes Journees Medicales Sur les Problemes Psychologiques en Rapport Avec le Cancer:* Marseille, France, 7, No. 12 (1977).

[31]C. M. Parkes, *Bereavement Studies of Grief in Adult Life* (London: Tavistock Publications, 1972).

[32]C. S. Lewis, *A Grief Observed* (London: Faber and Faber, 1961).

[33]E. Lindemann, "Symptomatology and Management of Acute Grief," *Journal of Psychiatry,* 101 (1944), 141-48.

Chapter Ten

Marriage and the Family in Whole-Person Medicine

Lewis Penhall Bird

The past decade has witnessed a growing interest in "wholistic health care." Theorists, clinicians and sponsors have joined under various auspices in launching centers where such care could be obtained. Where such clinicians or programs address themselves to the psychosocial determinants of health and disease, husband-wife and family dynamics frequently become part of the focus of attention. Those particular aspects of one's psychosocial environment will be the concern of this paper.

Ten years ago one of the clinicians foremost in urging modern medicine to consider the role the family plays in patient well-being was a Canadian family practitioner and academic professor, Ian R. McWhinney. He said: "We are beginning to recognize that diagnosis is incomplete unless it includes an assessment of the family, the environment and the personality of the patient in relation to the illness."[1] Deliberately employing Lewis Mumford's phrase calling for "the primacy of the person,"[2] McWhinney observed later that "to restore the primacy of the person, one needs a medicine that puts the person in all his wholeness in the center of the stage and does not separate the disease from the man, and the man from his environment—a medicine that makes technology firmly subservient to human values, and maintains a creative balance between generalist and specialist."[3]

Writing elsewhere, McWhinney urged that "we come to see illness in the context of the whole person and his environment. . . . It is only the complexity of modern life that makes it necessary to make the terms explicit."[4] Speaking of the format of the typical clinicopathological conference, McWhinney raised the question: "How often do we discuss the patient as a person—his feelings, his values, his life story, his relationships and the complex interaction between these and his disease?"[5] In part, he answered his own inquiry: "If we omit [these] matters from our discussions, then we transmit unconsciously the message that we think them unimportant."[6] For McWhinney and many others, caring for the whole person means assessing marital and family relationships as well as physiological and emotional mechanisms. For him, whole-person medicine is what modern family medicine is all about; the two are basically synonymous.[7] His concern to explore the psychosocial environment is commendable; it underscores the place of the family in modern *family* medicine. Whether whole-person medicine is essentially synonymous with contemporary family-medicine practice, however, remains to be more fully explored.

"Holistic" Medicine
A fascinating counterpoint to the understanding of whole-person medicine has been a burgeoning enterprise known especially in California as "holistic" medicine. About a year ago the business magazine *Forbes* reviewed for the knowledgeable layperson this recently developing phenomenon. The article suggested that it would be "the patient's responsibility to modify elements in his daily living that might be making him sick: his job, diet, sex life, family relationships."[8] Wherever holistic medicine might be interested in the relational dimensions of illness, an alliance might be forged between therapists who treat marriage and family problems and medical clinicians at some points in treatment for the larger benefit of the defined patient. What are the intentions of holistic medicine?

Although holistic medicine conferences have been held recently in Philadelphia[9] and Washington,[10] it has been largely out of California's avant-garde fermentations that most holistic innovations have come.[11] In various treatment centers there, traditional Western medicine may be combined with Eastern mysticism, acupuncture, biofeedback, Transcendental Meditation, Transactional Analysis, yoga, Est, Rolfing, Gestalt therapy, herbology, astrology, nutritional therapy, guided imagery, polarity massage or dream analysis. With some of these practices neither conventional medicine nor Christian therapists would have any strong objections; with other techniques serious reservations would be lodged. A Washington internist, Michael Halberstam, has voiced his disquiet: "Holism is so democratic, so all-accepting of unconventional healing, that it is hard to think of any system of belief, from snake-handling to chiropractory, that it would reject."[12]

Evidently, in an effort to replace individualistic-mechanistic notions of disease with an individualistic-metaphysical model, holistic practitioners may have succeeded only in replacing impersonal, organ-oriented medical care with an egoistic, do-it-yourself clinical smorgasbord which blends the conventional with the unconventional in random, self-service fashion. The enthusiasm with which some eclectic practitioners offer the fadistic, the bizarre or the unproven, merits care monitoring. Whether this kind of holistic healer becomes only a footnote to medical history or secures a foothold and even accreditation remains to be seen. Of the indiscriminate therapy sometimes urged from such quarters, a pointed caution from epidemiologist Walter O. Spitzer may apply: "If there is anyone more irritating to me than one assuming a holier-than-thou attitude, it is the one who assumes the more-holistic-than-thou stance."[13]

Efforts to broaden the diagnostic and treatment focus of the physician beyond a physiological system alone or beyond the individual in isolation, however, are commendable. Many criticisms have been leveled in recent years against health-care delivery systems and health-education programs which have concentrated on the individual to the exclusion of the environment. In a notable essay in *The New England Journal*

of Medicine's "Sounding Board" documenting health education's frequent inability to change behavior meaningfully,
Cohen and Cohen commented: "Simplistic, facile, individ-
ualistic solutions cannot produce meaningful change."[14]

In a lecture delivered last spring at the Baylor University
School of Medicine, physiologist Eugene D. Robin considered
the role of "Determinism and Humanism in Modern Medicine." After exploring why modern medicine has become
more diagnosis-oriented than person-centered, he concluded: "Thus, knee-jerk medicine, which provides routine
approaches to individual patients, is not really good medicine."[15] Robin then raised the question: "Is the answer to better patient care the superficial modification of some current
type of medical specialty or some new specialty that emphasizes patient care? The answer probably is no. If there is a
deep philosophical error in the way that medicine is practiced, then the solution is to alter the philosophical base."[16]

Probably few physicians have done more to alter or to
clarify the philosophical base of participants in this conference with regard to whole-person medicine than Paul Tournier. In *The Whole Person in a Broken World,* Tournier suggested that the contemporary emphasis on individualism
represents the "great plague of modern times, which plunges
man into dreadful solitude."[17] Writing that polemic against
fragmented medical care in a Swiss milieu over thirty years
ago, his voice has awakened countless health-care personnel
the world over to the more integrated potential of their art.
Affirming the insights of his colleague, Henri Mentha, Tournier quotes with approval Mentha's definition of whole-person medicine:

> The characteristic mark of the medicine of the person is
> the fact that it keeps its eye on the sick person with his body,
> with his mind, and with his spirit and not upon this or that
> practice, this system or that instrument. This medicine goes
> beyond physical medicine, without our being able to assign
> exact limits to it and without being able to foresee whom the
> physician may draw into collaboration in a given case.[18]

It is the idea of the family as collaborator in therapy that this paper seeks to explore.

The Family and the Patient

Before turning to various definitions of whole-person medicine which have been proposed, three brief reminders of clinical occasions where the therapeutic alliance of spouse and/or family members is already at work may be useful. Since whole-person medicine would include, in my judgment, both utilization of the family network and cultivation of spiritual insight, these examples are particularly compelling.

Since one of the contributors to this conference is a distinguished pioneer in the care of the terminally ill, only a few observations from the hospice movement merit mention here. In a lecture at the annual meeting of the Royal College of Physicians and Surgeons of Canada about a year ago, Balfour Mount enumerated six distinctive features of the Palliative Care Service at the Royal Victoria Hospital in Montreal. Two are relevant here. First, a central part of the program is the "treatment and care of the patient and the family as a unit."[19] Second, a major "concern for the patient's psychological, emotional and spiritual needs"[20] was outlined. In the hospice concept, including the family and meeting the psychological and spiritual needs of the patient are central concerns. Incidentally, of no small consequence has been the discovery that "hospice care is much less expensive than acute care hospitals."[21] One review of the hospice movement has called it "a humane, holistic approach to medical care that has great support among all elements of society."[22]

A second example of the therapeutic alliance between patient and family derives from one of the nation's most innovative programs seeking to respond to the current epidemic of teen-age pregnancy, the Adolescent Pregnancy Program at the Johns Hopkins Hospital in Balitmore.[23] That five-year-old program routinely draws in the parents of adolescents aged eleven to seventeen already enrolled. In the curriculum derived from the comprehensive prenatal health-care plan, one of the supporting principles defines the plan as "family oriented: the whole-life unit concept has been utilized in which adolescent fathers, parents, grandparents, boy/girl friends, siblings, and significant other persons participate in the program."[24] Further, the curriculum is "whole-person oriented: it is expected that adolescents will emerge with a balanced life-style, with self-esteem, and with a personal integration that places emphasis on the physiological, the psychological, the sociological, and the spiritual."[25] The spiritual dimension is perceived to provide guidance "that will aid adolescents in the development of values with particular reference to such human concerns as self-discipline, courage, consideration, fairness, love, honesty, self-sacrifice, service, responsibility and sharing."[26] As with the hospice movement, the inclusion of family members and nurture for the human spirit are both conceived to be as important as essential medical services.

A third preliminary illustration demonstrating the interrelationship between personal pathology and family orientations is sexual dysfunction therapy. It has become standard practice in sexual therapy to treat couples conjointly. Such a procedure underscores the assumption that the marital dyad merits as much evaluation and intervention as the sexual dysfunction. Masters and Johnson comment: "It should be emphasized that the Foundation's basic premise of therapy insists that, although both husband and wife in a sexually dysfunctional marriage are treated, the marital relationship is considered as the patient. Probably this concept is best expressed in the statement that sexual dysfunction is indeed a marital-unit problem, certainly never only a wife's or only a husband's personal concern."[27] Their experience with the use of female surrogate partners for dysfunctional males (now abandoned largely for medico-legal reasons) disclosed an interesting fact. For many males, though adequate sexual performance could be achieved with a professional surrogate, the dysfunction would recur on return home to their own partner. The use of surrogates was terminated on discovery that the relational aspects of one's experience were critically important to genital performance. Masters and Johnson's third book, *The Pleasure Bond,* addresses the concept that "mutual pleasure sets a seal on emotional commitment."[28]

Not every sexual dysfunction arises out of marital discord, but Helen Singer Kaplan has asserted that "clearly, pathological dyadic patterns which create destructive, alienating sexual systems exist in many instances. Frequently it is apparent that the transactions between the couple played a crucial role in the etiology of the sexual problem of one or both partners, and subsequently served to reinforce that problem."[29] Consequently, the therapeutic participation of both marital partners is indicated in outlining a treatment plan.

All three of these examples offer a clinical backdrop to two significant characteristics of whole-person medicine: (1) either the marital dyad or the family network become part of the therapeutic encounter; (2) interpersonal commitment, human values and spiritual insight constitute a crucial level of exploration and discovery in personal transformation. The inclusion of family members and the insight of spiritual values are already a part of medical care in certain specialized situations. Those themes may also compose the central core of what is distinctive of wholistic medicine.

Definitions of Whole-Person Medicine

We turn now to various definitions of whole-person medicine. We will focus on the role spouses or family members are perceived to bring to the health-care model. Since other chapters address the spiritual implications of such a philosophy of medicine, only occasional references will be made here to that important level of relationships and values. The two questions on which we will focus are: What is whole-person medicine? and How does the family figure in definitions of wholistic medicine?

The broadened redefinition of health offered years ago by the World Health Organization has already been referred to in this book. "Health is a state of complete physical, mental, and social well-being and not merely the absence of disease or infirmity."[30] One may infer that the social dimension in that definition includes family support systems even though such relationships are not explicitly mentioned.

A fascinating doctoral dissertation that sought to capture the central meaning of human personhood in the writings of theologians Paul Tillich, Karl Rahner and Martin Buber, sociologists Robert Bellah and Peter Berger, and psychologists Abraham Maslow and Erik Erikson was completed in 1973 at the Catholic University of America by Ruth Whitney.[31] Whitney identified only in the writings of sociologist Robert Bellah a strong correlation between family dynamics and an understanding of the person. Of special interest is her assessment of Bellah's position: "The family's primary functions are pattern maintenance and tension management in the socialization process. The family's concern is 'the management of personality tensions that have their origin in needs with an organic substratum.' "[32] Such an insight has clinical as well as philosophical implications. Whitney's study failed to locate any other perspectives correlating themes in family dynamics with understandings of our common humanity, although it is possible that such associations could be uncovered in the writings of those seven theorists.

In Bellah's understanding of family functions, "pattern maintenance" could have implications for personal homeostasis and "tension management" could have meaning for personal healing. Certainly such extrapolations are not inherently excluded. Also, Bellah's concern for the organic substratum will have appeal for wholistic-medicine practitioners whose roots are embedded in conventional medical strategies.

For specific correlations between health care and the family unit, consider a 1960 paper on "A Holistic Approach in the Management of Angina Pectoris." That approach was defined as "establishing satisfactory rapport with the patient, assisting in job placement, establishment of correct attitudes toward the job, offering reassurance, encouragement of frequent office visits, lessening family tension and prescribing tranquilizers rather than vasodilators."[33] It is interesting to note that family dynamics were presumed to be negatively skewed.

A 1963 study on "Talking with Doctors in Urbanville" compared comprehensive physicians with constricted doctors. The former had "a comprehensive role concept, accepting social perceptions and an open system of medical beliefs and values."[34] "Social perceptions" included family interactions.

In dissertation research on "A Study of the Holistic Approach in Primary Care," Moira Stewart discovered that the terms *comprehensive* and *holistic* are not necessarily used interchangeably: "In general, writers who referred to such matters as the team approach or continuity used the term comprehensive care, whereas writers who talked about the doctor-patient relationship tended to use the term holistic care."[35] That note of clarification may be helpful.

For her research purposes, Stewart defined holistic care as: care which took account of the patient's physical, psychological and social problems. In other words, the physician viewed the patient's mind, body and environment as integral parts of his being and all these parts were taken into account in the physician's data-gathering and management. . . . A further feature of the definition of holistic care in this research, in addition to the importance of physical, psychological and social factors presented by the patient, was the consideration of the impact or implications of these factors on the daily life of the patient.[36]

In that definition, the family may be presumed to be part of the social or environmental milieu since in the questionnaire used in Stewart's study to elicit specific psychosocial problems, relationships with spouse and with children were included in the list of topics to be assessed.[37]

Granger Westberg inaugurated wholistic health centers in the Midwest during the early 1970s; his influence in defining that particular kind of medical care cannot be overlooked:

In treatment as well as philosophy, whole person health care uses a wide angle lens to view the complex health concerns people bring to us, exploring the emotional, spiritual, intellectual, social and lifestyle issues as well as physical symptoms in facilitating health. . . . The basic starting premise for a wholistic view of health is that the individual is an integrated whole, with each dimension (physical, emotional, intellectual, social, spiritual) inextricably bound up with the whole.[38]

Again the social parameter may be construed to include family dynamics; a later statement affirms that "friends, family, a sense of community, as well as religious faith, a sense of purpose in life, and personal commitments are all taken seriously and considered important in the fostering of the healing process."[39]

Health-care providers in the nursing community have used the phrase *whole-person medicine* for several years now. Myra E. Levine relates "holistic nursing" to four patient parameters: energy, structural integrity, personal integrity and social integrity. The family figures in the latter:

> Every individual is defined by his social group, and often the integrity of the patient is intimately interwoven in the fabric of his cultural, ethnic, religious, and family relationships. . . . The holistic view of the individual must include the close, personal ties he has with his life beyond the predicament of illness itself. Individual well-being is always a portion of a collective well-being, and the isolation of patienthood does not terminate the essential interactions and dependencies which family members have with one another. The families of hospitalized patients are frequently left outside the circle of concern.[40]

One might add that the family dynamics of outpatients are frequently overlooked as well.

Clearly, the husband-wife relationship and the family network are explicitly or implicitly subsumed in various definitions of whole-person medicine.

Some Biblical Considerations

Two generations of theologians have debated whether persons are to be perceived as two-part beings (body, spirit) or as three-part beings (body, soul, spirit). Do biblical and theological roots provide a substantial conceptual foundation for the contemporary emphasis on whole-person medicine? As we shall see, theologians today typically speak more of Hebraic wholism than of either dichotomy or trichotomy.

The effort to construct a biblical anthropology has engaged theological minds for centuries. Part of the difficulty arises from the fact that "psychological functions are attributed to the eye, ear, mouth, flesh, bones, belly, breast, loins, and thighs"[41] and the fact that Hebrew words for soul *(nephesh)*, spirit *(ruach)* and heart *(leb)* are used either interchangeably or with such subtle differences that psychological boundaries are impossible to construct. The dilemma led John A. T. Robinson to comment: "From the standpoint of analytic psychology and physiology the usage of the Old Testament is chaotic: it is the nightmare of the anatomist when any part can stand at any moment for the whole and similar functions be predicated of such various organs as the heart, the kidneys and the bowels—not to mention the soul."[42]

Such observations led H. Wheeler Robinson to his now famous aphorism, "The Hebrew idea of the personality is an animated body, and not an incarnated soul."[43] Writing in 1925, Robinson acknowledged that "there is no trichotomy in Hebrew psychology, no triple division of human personality into 'body, soul, and spirit.' "[44] Old Testament scholar Walter Eichrodt echoed that conclusion. *Nephesh* and *ruach,* he wrote, "always represent the whole life of the person from a particular point of view. A trichotomistic human psychology is therefore as little to be based on the Old Testament concepts as a dualistic one."[45]

Assumptions about dichotomy in the New Testament writings based on Greek dualism have received significant censure. Philologist James Barr cautioned: "There are difficulties and snags in the use of the Hebrew-Greek contrast."[46] Arguments for dualism in the ante-Nicene or post-Nicene fathers may derive more from either Platonic or Gnostic influences than from any Judeo-Christian canonical writings. Reflecting on Pauline psychology, George Ladd affirms more recent scholarship which recognizes the familiar terms of body, soul and spirit to be but "different ways of viewing the whole man."[47]

Following a review of biblical data, distinguished Reformed scholar G. C. Berkouwer concluded: "It appears clearly, then, that Scripture never pictures man as a dualistic, or pluralistic being, but that in all its varied expressions the whole man comes to the fore, in all his guilt and sin, his need and oppression, his longings and his nostalgia."[48] A similar conclusion was reached in the recently released Christian Association for Psychological Studies monograph by David G. Myers: "The holistic image implied by the resurrection doctrine is deeply consistent with the holistic anthropology of the Old and New Testaments—and with the emerging scientific picture as well."[49]

This insight has practical implications for individuals identified with the Judeo-Christian tradition and interested in whole-person medicine. From even a cursory review of the concept of Hebraic wholism, several conclusions merit consideration:

1. Holding an antiquated view of human personhood, whether dichotomous or trichotomous, may make it easier for Christian health practitioners to justify diagnostic and treatment plans whereby only a certain segment of an individual's disequilibrium is served. Such a rationale, ignoring recent and responsible biblical scholarship, may permit clinicians, perhaps subconsciously, to treat the part with little concern for the whole, thus perpetuating one of the major problems that health-care consumers have come to decry.

2. Adoption of a unitary view of human personhood by health-care practitioners in the Judeo-Christian tradition could give wholistic care special appeal. That philosophy of medicine does not necessarily imply that a single individual would have to be the sole health-care provider nor that medical specialists would be excluded.

3. If a wholistic view of human personhood when related to health-care delivery systems is perceived to imply that multilevel investigations should accompany every patient interview, whether presenting with acute or chronic complaints and whether the visit be for routine insurance exams, booster shots or children's checkups, then the costs, manpower and time required could reach astronomical proportions. Obviously, some selection criteria and management strategies are

needed if the assumption warrants clinical implementation. And if traditional religious understandings of human nature, which segmented functions into physiological, emotional and spiritual parts, provided clearly defined boundaries in the past for ministry, surely a recovered Hebraic wholism will have innovative implications for some sectors of the health-care community both in the present and in the future.

Another refinement in understanding the possibilities of wholistic health care from a religious point of view proceeds from exploration of Hebraic and Christian roots. Since the present essay focuses on the relationship between whole-person medicine and marriage and the family, one cannot over-look the biblical notion of *henosis:* the unity derived from the "one flesh" experience in marriage.[50] Anglican theologian Derrick Sherwin Bailey devoted a whole book to a considera-tion of henosis, his *Mystery of Love and Marriage.*[51] "Although the union in 'one flesh' is a physical union established by sexual intercourse (the conjunction of the sexual organs), it involves at the same time the whole being, and affects the per-sonality at the deepest level. It is a union of the entire man and the entire woman. In it they become a new and distinct unity, wholly different from and set over against other human relational unities."[52]

Otto Piper's study *The Biblical View of Sex and Marriage* de-fined the "one flesh" henosis as "a unity that embraces the natural lives of the two persons in their entirety"[53] thereby creating "mutual dependence and reciprocity in all areas of life."[54] Bailey and Piper explored henosis in relation to mar-riage and sexuality without calling attention to the other end of the pleasure-pain spectrum: henosis in relation to human suffering. Bailey made the provocative statement, however, that "the henosis of man and woman, each the diametrical opposite of the other, is the symbol of what love could do toward the healing of those divisions from which humanity and the Church suffer so grievously."[55]

The "one flesh" meaning of henosis is vested with multiple metaphysical implications for the covenantally committed. One cannot avoid raising questions about its relevance for

212   Whole-Person Medicine

the couple coping with trauma or disease processes. The wholistic concept argues that Mrs. Brown rather than "the mastectomy in room 541" should be treated. Does not the henosis concept urge medical personnel to care for both Mrs. and Mr. Brown as they jointly come to terms with that mastectomy?

In other words, in what particular circumstances can the henotic relationship be enlisted in the healing process? On what occasions can a henotic relationship contribute to or be enlisted in vigorous preventative programs? Without necessarily being theologically inclined, Masters and Johnson soon recognized the necessity of including both marital partners in any sexual dysfunction therapy. The henotic union in a marital dyad does not merely consummate a marriage; it also either confirms a deeper covenantal communion than language will ever be able to describe fully or it defines the battleground around which a larger and more destructive war can devastate an intimate relationship. Modern medical care should not overlook the enormous strength found in healthy marital relationships. As Karl Barth noted, "In the battle against sickness the final human word cannot be isolation but only fellowship."[56]

Having assessed how marital and family relationships are included in some definitions of whole-person medicine, having reviewed briefly the recovery of Hebraic wholism in the construction of a biblical anthropology, and having touched on the implications the biblical notion of henosis may have for treating married adults, we now turn to the interrelationship between family support systems and personal health dysfunctions.

Family Support Systems and Personal Health Dysfunction
Although correlations between personal health and family life have come increasingly to the fore in the investigations of family-medicine clinicians, that linkage has not always been a focus of attention. From the ancillary perspective of pediatrics and child care, I. B. Pless and B. Satterwhite in 1975 concluded that "one of the most important aspects of pediatrics is

the emphasis placed on the family unit. Few child health workers would deny that the quality of family life is closely related to the health of children. Nevertheless, remarkably little attention has been paid to the family as an object of systematic study by those interested in medical care research."[57]

The predictive ability of correlating family dynamics with individual health patterns is evident, however, in one of the early pediatric studies designed to investigate such correlations, the Meyer and Haggerty study on "Streptococcal Infections in Families."[58] When the family environment was monitored "by means of the interview [method] and diaries, life events that disrupted family or personal life and caused excess anxiety, and other evidences of disorganization were independently recorded."[59] Part of the findings were that:

about one quarter of the streptococcal acquisitions and illnesses followed such acute family crises, and there was an even clearer relation between both acquisitions and illness and these acute crises when the period 2 weeks before and 2 weeks after acquisitions or illness was compared.... Streptococcal acquisition and illness, as well as non-streptococcal respiratory infections, were about four times as likely to be preceded as to be followed by acute stress.... An equally useful dependent variable was the level of chronic stress found in each family.[60]

The correlation of respiratory infections with acute family stress was noted in conjunction with such factors as the loss of a family member, serious illness in another family member, a minor illness with serious complications, a nonmedical family crisis, a nonfamily crisis and multiple family stresses.

The Meyer and Haggerty study can be seen as a fascinating precursor to the better-known Holmes and Rahe Social Readjustment Rating Scale.[61] In that inventory, stressful life events associated with varying amounts of disruption in the average person's life were given weighted scores on an impact scale. Those scores became known as "Life Change Units"; an accumulation of 200 or more LCUs in a single year could be predictive for most Americans of the common stress diseases. Six out of the ten highest-scoring events have to do with family matters: death of a spouse, divorce, marital separation, death of a close family member, getting married, marital reconciliation. The remaining four high-scoring events have obvious family implications: receiving a jail term, personal injury or illness, getting fired at work, retirement. If whole-person medicine includes assessing marital and family dynamics, then certain individual patients would be treated in the clear context of their social environment rather than only symptomatically.

The research of Friedman and Rosenman regarding "Type A" behavior and heart disease represents another correlation of lifestyle, coping mechanisms and family dynamics with disease processes.[62] The interrelationship between premature death from coronary heart disease and family dislocation has been amply documented by James Lynch. He concluded: "The fact is that social isolation, the lack of human companionship, death or absence of parents in early childhood, sudden loss of love, and chronic human loneliness are significant contributors to premature death."[63]

Regimens that specifically incorporated family dynamics as part of the treatment plan have been directed toward angina pectoris,[64] multiple sclerosis,[65] and rheumatoid arthritis.[66] In an admirable review of the literature on "The Family as The Unit of Medical Care," David D. Schmidt considered the thesis that "when providing primary medical care, there seems to be a definite advantage in centering this care about the family unit rather than the isolated individual patient."[67] His first category, "The Family's Contribution to the 'Cause' of Disease," reviewed relevant studies on upper respiratory tract infection, streptococcal infections, stroke susceptibility, pregnancy complications, tuberculosis, malignant neoplasms, arteriosclerotic heart disease and three psychiatric problems: sociopathic personality disorder, suicide and depression.

A second category examined "The Family's Contribution to the 'Cure' of Disease"; studies in rehabilitation with stroke victims, severe orthopedic disabilities, alcoholism, heart disease and rheumatoid arthritis along with patient medication compliance were noted. In the category, "The Family's Response to Serious or Chronic Disease," studies reviewed considered modifications in family dynamics caused by the sick role of the patient in coping with diabetes, hemophilia, hypertensive vascular disease, total circulatory disease and arthritis. The fourth category, "The Family's Desire and/or Need for Family-Oriented Care," described those studies which identified particular families where intensive, comprehensive, family-centered care might be especially indicated.

In an effort to provide the clinician with a diagnostic device sensitive to family dynamics, in 1972 McWhinney proposed "A Taxonomy of Social Factors in Illness and in Patient Behavior" to be derived from current life situations and which could be amenable to alteration. His seven categories were (1) Loss, personal or possessions; (2) Conflict, interpersonal or intrapersonal; (3) Change, developmental or geographic; (4) Maladjustment, interpersonal or personal; (5) Stress, acute or chronic; (6) Isolation; and (7) Failure or frustrated expectations.[68] A year later Pless published a sixteen-item, self-administered questionnaire on family functioning which assessed such issues as communication, problem solving, frequency of disagreements, marital satisfaction and weekends together.[69] A five-year follow-up study demonstrated its reliability as a predictor of family dysfunction.[70]

In epidemiologist Moira Stewart's study of a wholistic approach in primary care, thirteen chronic illnesses served as criteria for the entry of patients into the investigation. Those illnesses were obesity, chronic hypertension, chronic bronchitis and asthma, varicose veins, congestive heart failure, other heart ailments, diabetes, chronic arthritis, chronic back pain, ischemic heart disease, chronic ulcer, chronic skin condition and stroke.[71] Those conditions were selected by a panel of clinicians on the basis of their relatively high frequency in a primary-care practice.[72] Stewart then posited eleven indicators of wholistic care:

1. Knowledge of complaints
2. Awareness of patient's concept

3. Knowledge of magnitude of discomfort
4. Knowledge of magnitude of worry
5. Knowledge of magnitude of disturbance of daily living
6. Knowledge of existence of social problems
7. Knowledge of magnitude of social problems
8. Response to discomfort
9. Response to worry
10. Response to disturbance of daily living
11. Response to social problems.[73]

The Stewart study represents one of the first efforts to approach wholistic medicine rigorously, with evaluation predicated on measurable indices. Regrettably, assessing whether or not whole-person care made any perceptible difference to the patient's outcome was beyond demonstration. Four reasons were offered in explanation: imperfections of the outcome measurements; reservations about the accuracy of the indicators of wholistic care as measures of the process of care; the confounding effect of other factors; and the lag-time between care and effect.[74] Further research will be needed in evaluation measurements if whole-person medicine is to be validated in various medical settings.

Systems Theory

One final theme merits brief exploration: how can an understanding of systems theory relate concerns about family dynamics to whole-person medicine? Two definitions are in order. Von Bertalanffy defined a system as "a dynamic order of parts and processes standing in mutual interaction."[75] In Waller's words, family dynamics describes the "unity of personalities acting upon one another."[76] That interaction of personalities in a systematic way concerns us here.

Incidentally, the only reference to *holism* indexed in the recently released *Encyclopedia of Bioethics* is directed to Savodnik's discussion of biological systems. In his words, "holism asserts that the organization of biological systems is what distinguishes them from nonliving systems, and hence, in a manner of speaking, the whole of the living system is greater than the sum of its parts."[77] The appeal of wholism derives from its congruence with sound scientific principles, its affirmation of human freedom and its openness to moral responsibility. Savodnik considers one's response to biological reductionism especially crucial to the ethical problems of the sanctity of life, abortion, euthanasia and genetic engineering.

An additional insight derives from the work of neo-Freudian psychoanalyst and theoretician, Karen Horney. In Meissner's words, "she formulated a holistic notion of the personality as an individual unit functioning within a social framework and continually caught up in interaction and mutual influence with its environment. While she recognized the role of biological needs and drives, she shifted the emphasis in her theory of personality and neurosis to the dynamic influences of cultural and social factors."[78] Such an effort to discern personality development in the matrix of family dynamics and with a wholistic perspective can contribute further insight to our theme.

Scanzoni and Scanzoni provide a helpful review of the five basic frameworks within which family dynamics are usually assessed.[79] Although three of those perspectives (the developmental framework, conflict theory and the social exchange framework) provide only marginal insights relevant to family dynamics in whole-person medicine, the remaining two offer quite attractive perspectives. The first of these, the interactional framework, focuses attention on the internal dynamics operating within the family unit itself. Bonding and communication processes, role playing, behavioral actions and reactions provide the vistas from which interactions can be understood. In that view, communication theory and action-reaction responses would be of vital interest to any wholistic-medicine clinician.[80]

The other relevant framework is the structure-functional perspective, which emphasizes the family as a social system. Building on the work in systems theory of Bertalanffy and Buckley,[81] structure-functional family theorists emphasize both order and equilibrium in family relationships. In the words of the Scanzonis, "this framework uses the analogy of the human body with all its interdependent parts having specific functions to perform in order to maintain the steady-state condition of good health."[82] In this view, the focus is upon family function. The tensions and conflicts that disrupt the homeostasis or equilibrium of the individual family member become the object of inquiry and intervention. That understanding of family dynamics concerns itself with system maintenance and speaks of family experiences according to their functional or dysfunctional effects.

One discovers in family dynamics perceived as a special kind of social system an attractive format for health-care personnel seeking to establish a practice of whole-person medicine. Physicians particularly are trained already to think of physical systems, but whole-person medicine concerns the social milieu as well. Since physicians diagnose already with reference to the cardiovascular system, the pulmonary system, the renal, metabolic, endocrine, gastrointestinal, central nervous, reproductive and muscular-skeletal systems, the present essay proposes that physicians seek to diagnose with reference to the family system also. Since the negative correlation between family dynamics and personal dysfunction, and the positive connection between disease processes and responsive family actions, are already well known, definitive inquiries probing the patient's family interactions could be productive.

In order to understand family interactions in a systems manner, consider for a moment how family dynamics might be perceived as an integrated endocrine system (I am indebted to Janet Seely of the McGill University faculty at the Kellogg Centre for Advanced Studies in Primary Care for this insightful analogy).[83] In the endocrine system homeostasis is preserved through the proper function of the cortex, hypothalamus, pituitary and thyroid, parathyroid, pancreatic and adrenal glands as well as the male or female gonads. At least three relevant observations may be made about the endocrine system: the system is usually in balance; in considering the operation of the system, the focus is on interrelationships of hormones; and in assessing pathology, the symptomatology may be in several places at once, with symptoms distant from the original site of disturbance.

In an analogy relating family dynamics to the endocrine system, if the cortex is thought of as one's ancestors, if the hypothalamus is seen as the grandparents, if the pituitary is understood as parental control and if the various other glands are perceived as the children in a family, then the same three observations can be made of the family as a system: the system has its own kind of balance; in considering any dysfunction, the focus is on interrelationships; and in assessing family pathology, the symptomatology may be in several persons at the same time and the various manifestations may be quite removed from the precipitating source.

For example, one child with severe stomach pains is seen by a pediatrician while a sibling is scheduled to see the school counselor because her work is far below capabilities. Meanwhile, the father is being treated by his internist for gastric ulcers, whereupon it is discovered that the mother has just begun full-time graduate studies for her master's degree in a family where finances are tight, marital conflict is common and a home-cooked meal is presumed to be necessary every evening. Whole-person medicine would be as concerned with family systems as with the gastrointestinal tract.

Conclusions

1. For those particularly committed to a Judeo-Christian reference point, recovery of the Hebraic heritage of wholistic anthropology could provide a viable conceptual foundation from which to construct programs of whole-person medicine.

2. For those committed both to understanding and supporting the institution of marriage, explorations beyond merely the symbolic level of meaning in the "one flesh" henotic union could possibly lend clearer perspective to the range of marital function and dysfunction inherent in that intimacy.

3. Since physicians are accustomed to patient examination, diagnosis and treatment organized around various physiological systems, evaluating certain patients with reference to the family system could provide a natural motif for assessing personal dysfunction. Accordingly, health-care personnel

at various levels will need to acquaint themselves with such a systems analysis. Some post-graduate educational programs for physicians are already moving in that direction.[84] In my view, the incorporation of such an approach to the clinical management of patient problems would be one crucial element in defining whole-person medicine.

4. It may be appropriate to devise selection criteria that could indicate which specific problems or occasions merit a family systems analysis more clearly than others. To evaluate marital and/or family relationships during an immunization program or following trauma or in the treatment of an acute health problem may not be warranted. Unbridled enthusiasm for wholistic medicine could lead to excesses at the outset which ultimately could prove deleterious to a potentially admirable philosophy of medicine.

5. Too broad a definition of whole-person medicine could consume inordinate amounts of time, money and clinical energy if the physician must perceive himself or herself to be not only doctor to the patient but chaperone, financial adviser, social director and fishing companion as well. Paul Ramsey has expressed legitimate concern over the moral implications that allegiance to the World Health Organization's definition of health as general human "well-being" could have. Consistently applied, such a practice "would be to locate medical considerations in direct lineage with all of man's moral reflection upon the meaning of *eudaimonia* (well-being, happiness) since Aristotle!"[85]

6. Too narrow a definition of whole-person medicine could permit health-care providers to dismiss family relationships or considerations of personal lifestyle in good conscience after only a casual inquiry. Theodore Lidz's remarkable study, *The Person,* is a common text for seminars on whole-person medicine; after the preface he has a special section entitled, "Remarks to the Reader—If a Medical Student."[86] His observations address a narrow-minded concept of medical care. Lidz suggests that among the motivations for studying medicine "there must be an interest in people and a desire to help them, a wish to stand with the patient against his fate

and help him avert tragedy, and when one cannot, to help provide the strength to bear it. If there is no such interest in people, a student cannot properly become a physician. He can still become a medical scientist, for which there is great need, and become very helpful to mankind, but not a physician."[87]

7. Exploring personal values which contribute directly to lifestyle could be a compelling part of whole-person medicine. Although little attention has been directed in this chapter to the spiritual dimension of whole-person medicine, that aspect of patient care will be an obvious concern of Christian physicians. Increasing support can be found in the literature for considering the spiritual dimension of life as inherently included in health care. In the judgment of health educator Harold J. Cornacchia, "probably the most important influence on health, yet the one most frequently overlooked or omitted in teaching, is the spiritual aspect."[88] Further, although insistent voices have cautioned, legitimately, against imposing personal values on patients, little creative imagination seems to have been expended on the possibilities of either sharing or eliciting personal values in meaningful circumstances.

8. How a physician might enter more fully into the patient's experience has been discussed by many of us over the years. A frequent anxiety concerns either the inordinate amount of time such inquiry might take or the neurotic mechanisms which might be triggered in the so-called crocks of life. With regard to time constraints, an imaginative cultivation of therapeutic one-liners could provide numerous balms in Gilead in place of either avoidance syndromes or professional small talk. Special strategies are outlined in James E. Grove's analysis of what he calls the "hateful patient" (that is, "dependent clingers," "entitled demanders," "manipulative help-rejecters," and "self-destructive deniers").[89]

Many challenges face the advocate of whole-person medicine. Every cliché has its day. Evidence on outcomes for wholistic medicine is only beginning to be gathered. For the single person, an assessment of the meaningful other persons in their lives might be indicated. Only when substantive gains can be documented will careful clinicians find wholistic medicine more than a bandwagon slogan. And if whole-person medicine does prove to be the royal road to cost-efficient, patient-benefiting, health-care delivery, efficient ways of teaching its strategy to already overburdened clinicians in a technologically explosive career will need to be found.

Earlier we discovered that Hebraic understandings of wholism have particular relevance to whole-person medicine. A growing audience is beginning to appreciate the linguistic interrelationships between health, wholeness and salvation.[90] A cognate in that family of words is the Hebrew blessing, *shalom*. In a classic study, Pedersen discovered in *shalom* not only the absence of strife, but also "the fact of being whole and he who is whole."[91] Gerhard von Rad found the root meaning to be " 'well-being,' with a strong emphasis on the material side."[92] In various biblical examples, bodily health is intended.[93] Perhaps the larger view of *shalom* was best captured by J. Barton Payne. Not only is a "state of integration"[94] implied, but "this term carries with it, positively, the rich implications of soundness and wholeness, of that full integration of life which becomes possible only for those who live in tune with the One who is the Master of all that a man may encounter."[95]

Perhaps whole-person medicine will signal the advent of a more sensitive kind of medical care grounded in the concept of *shalom*.

Afterword

Whether one's world view is primarily theological or philosophical, the traditional dichotomous, trichotomous, or Cartesian dualistic efforts to construct a useful clinical anthropology may seem obsolete (Figure 10.1). A valuable critique of the Cartesian understanding of the nature of human persons, especially as it affects issues in biomedical ethics, is found in the recently released Macmillan *Encyclopedia of Bioethics*.

A potentially more useful index for practicing whole-person medicine might be to recognize the multifaceted

Figure 10.1 Traditional Models of Anthropology

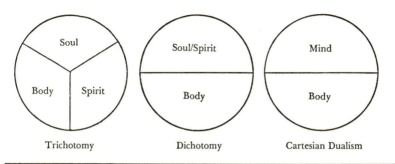

Trichotomy · Dichotomy · Cartesian Dualism

dimensions of human personhood in a schema which uses modern terms more clearly understood and less encumbered with the traditional debates (which frequently fail to persuade contemporary minds). This motif (Figure 10.2) permits the clinician to have in view both the traditional medical aspects of

Figure 10.2 Contemporary Understanding of Human Personhood

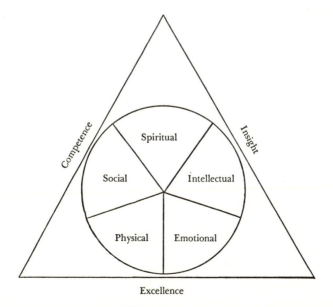

patient care for which he or she has been trained to inter-
cede and the other major components of patient life with
which the doctor may need to interject aid. The cultivation
of additional skills or the development of a referral system
which turns to other trained professionals could provide the
mechanisms for treatment once the clinician assumes a wholistic approach in practice.

In this view traditional medical skills would be practiced
with excellence, some competence in assessing marital or family and spiritual dynamics would be acquired, and insight regarding the patient's ability to perceive both mentally and
spiritually the nature of their problem would be included in
the treatment plan.

Notes

[1]Ian R. McWhinney, "Advances in General Practice," *The Practitioner*, 203 (October 1969), 535-40.

[2]Lewis Mumford, *The Condition of Man* (New York: Harcourt, Brace and World, 1944).

[3]Ian R. McWhinney, "Family Medicine in Perspective," *New England Journal of Medicine*, 293, No. 4 (24 July 1975), 176-81.

[4]Ian R. McWhinney, "Continuity of Care in Family Practice," *Journal of Family Practice*, 2, No. 5 (1975), 373-74.

[5]Ian R. McWhinney, "Medicine as an Art Form," *Canadian Medical Association Journal*, 114 (24 January 1976), 98-101.

[6]Ibid.

[7]Personal phone conversation, 25 January 1979.

[8]*Forbes*, 120, No. 7 (1 October 1977), 44.

[9]The Philadelphia conference, "Holistic Perspectives: a Renaissance in Medicine and Health Care," was sponsored by the Institute for Holistic Health and Education and the Hahnemann Medical College in November 1978 with approximately 700 attending.

[10]Compare Michael Halberstam, "Holistic Healing: Limits of 'The New Medicine,' " *Psychology Today*, 12, No. 3 (August 1978), 26-27.

[11]Compare *Forbes* (1 October 1977); *San José Mercury News* (8 April 1978), Section C, pp. 1ff.

[12]Halberstam, p. 26.

[13]Walter O. Spitzer, "Issues for Team Delivery and Interdisciplinary Education: A Canadian Perspective," *Journal of Medical Education*, 50, Part 2 (1975), 117-21.

[14]Carl I. Cohen and Ellen J. Cohen, "Health Education: Panacea, Pernicious or Pointless?" *New England Journal of Medicine*, 299, No. 13 (28 September 1978), 718-20.

[15]Eugene D. Robin, "Determinism and Humanism in Modern Medicine,"

Journal of the American Medical Association, 240, No. 21 (17 November 1978), 2273-75.

[16]Ibid.

[17]Paul Tournier, *The Whole Person in a Broken World,* trans. John and Helen Doberstein (New York: Harper & Row, 1964), p. 157.

[18]Ibid., p. 64.

[19]Balfour M. Mount, "Palliative Care of the Terminally Ill," *Annals of the Royal College of Physicians and Surgeons of Canada* (July 1978), 201-8.

[20]Ibid.

[21]William M. Markel and Virginia B. Sinon, "The Hospice Concept," *CA-A Cancer Journal for Clinicians,* 28, No. 4 (July/August 1978), 225-37.

[22]Ibid.

[23]Eunice Kennedy Shriver, "A Surprising View of Teen-Age Pregnancy," *Ladies' Home Journal,* 95, No. 11 (November 1978), 100ff.

[24]Denese A. Shipp, Lewis Penhall Bird and Harold J. Cornacchia, *Caring for the Pregnant Adolescent: Teacher's Manual* (New York: Doubleday, in press), chap. 7, "The Curriculum."

[25]Ibid.

[26]Ibid.

[27]William H. Masters and Virginia E. Johnson, *Human Sexual Inadequacy* (Boston: Little, Brown and Co., 1970), p. 3.

[28]William H. Masters and Virginia E. Johnson, *The Pleasure Bond: A New Look at Sexuality and Commitment* (Boston: Little, Brown and Co., 1975), p. 253.

[29]Helen Singer Kaplan, *The New Sex Therapy* (New York: Brunner/Mazel, 1974), p. 236.

[30]Cited in James B. Nelson, *Rediscovering the Person in Medical Care* (Minneapolis: Augsburg Publishing House, 1976), p. 24.

[31]Ruth Whitney, "An Understanding of Person in the Tillichian Dialectic and Its Implications for Women in American Society: An Interdisciplinary Study," Diss. Catholic University of America, Washington, D.C., 1973.

[32]Ibid., p. 347.

[33]I. S. Eskwith, "A Holistic Approach in the Management of Angina Pectoris," *Postgraduate Medicine,* 27 (1960), 203-6.

[34]S. Wolfe, "Talking with Doctors in Urbanville: An Exploratory Study of Canadian General Practitioners," *American Journal of Public Health,* 53 (1963), 631-44.

[35]Moira Anne Stewart, "A Study of the Holistic Approach in Primary Care," Diss. University of Western Ontario, 1975, p. 8.

[36]Ibid., pp. 29, 32.

[37]Ibid., p. 181.

[38]Nancy Loving Tubesing, *Whole Person Health Care: Philosophical Assumptions* (Hinsdale, Ill.: Wholistic Health Centers, Inc., 1977), p. 5.

[39]Ibid., p. 25.

[40]Myra E. Levine, "The Four Conservation Principles of Nursing," handout at the Second Annual Nurse Educator Conference (New York City, December 1978); see also her "Wholistic Nursing," *Nursing Clinics of North America,* 6 (June 1971), 253-64.

[41]David G. Myers, *The Human Puzzle: Psychological Research and Christian*

Belief (New York: Harper & Row, 1978), p. 75.

[42]John A. T. Robinson, *The Body: A Study in Pauline Theology* (London: SCM Press, 1952), p. 16.

[43]H. Wheeler Robinson, "Hebrew Psychology," in *The People and the Book,* ed. A. S. Peake (New York: Oxford University Press, 1925), p. 362.

[44]Ibid.

[45]Walter Eichrodt, *Theology of the Old Testament,* trans. J. A. Baker (Philadelphia: Westminster Press, 1967), II, 148.

[46]James Barr, *The Semantics of Biblical Language* (London: Oxford University Press, 1961), p. 20. See chapter 2, "The Current Contrast of Greek and Hebrew Thought."

[47]George Eldon Ladd, *A Theology of the New Testament* (Grand Rapids, Mich.: Eerdmans, 1974), p. 457. See his chapter 33, "The Pauline Psychology." Ladd agrees with Whiteley's "modification of the unitary view" of human personhood in the face of the Pauline sense of survival of the self following death, without succumbing either to dichotomy or trichotomy. See pp. 463-64.

[48]G. C. Berkouwer, *Man: The Image of God,* trans. Dirk W. Jellema (Grand Rapids, Mich.: Eerdmans, 1962), p. 203.

[49]Myers, p. 86.

[50]Gen. 2:24; Mt. 19:5; 1 Cor. 6:16; Eph. 5:31.

[51]Derrick Sherwin Bailey, *Mystery of Love and Marriage* (New York: Harper and Brothers, 1952).

[52]Ibid., p. 28.

[53]Otto A. Piper, *The Biblical View of Sex and Marriage* (New York: Charles Scribner's Sons, 1960), p. 25.

[54]Ibid., p. 28.

[55]Bailey, p. 116.

[56]Karl Barth, *Church Dogmatics,* trans. A. T. Mackay et al. (Edinburgh: T. & T. Clark, 1961), III, Part 4, 363.

[57]I. B. Pless and B. Satterwhite, "Family Functioning and Family Problems," in *Child Health and the Community,* ed. R. J. Haggerty, K. J. Roghman and I. B. Pless (New York: John Wiley and Sons, 1975), p. 41.

[58]Roger J. Meyer and Robert J. Haggerty, "Streptococcal Infections in Families," *Pediatrics,* 29, No. 4 (April 1962), 539-49.

[59]Ibid.

[60]Ibid.

[61]R. H. Holmes and R. H. Rahe, "The Social Readjustment Rating Scale," *Journal of Psychosomatic Research,* 11 (1967), 213-18.

[62]Meyer Friedman and Ray H. Rosenman, *Type A Behavior and Your Heart* (New York: Alfred A. Knopf, 1974).

[63]James J. Lynch, *The Broken Heart: The Medical Consequences of Loneliness* (New York: Basic Books, 1977), p. 3.

[64]Eskwith, pp. 203-6.

[65]Michael F. Hartings, Marcia M. Pavlou and Floyd A. Davis, "Group Counseling of MS Patients in a Program of Comprehensive Care," *Journal of Chronic Disease,* 29 (1976), 65-73.

[66]S. Katz et al., "Comprehensive Outpatient Care in Rheumatoid Arthritis: A Controlled Study," *Journal of the American Medical Association,* 206

(1968), 1249-54.

[67]David D. Schmidt, "The Family as the Unit of Medical Care," *Journal of Family Practice*, 7, No. 2 (1978), 303-13.

[68]Ian R. McWhinney, "Beyond Diagnosis: An Approach to the Integration of Behavioral Science and Clinical Medicine," *New England Journal of Medicine*, 287, No. 8 (24 August 1972), 384-87.

[69]I. B. Pless and B. B. Satterwhite, "A Measure of Family Functioning and Its Application," *Social Science and Medicine*, 7 (1973), 613ff.

[70]B. B. Satterwhite et al., "The Family Functioning Index: Five-year Test/ Retest Reliability and Implications for Use," *Journal of Comparative Family Studies*, 7 (1976), 111 ff.

[71]Stewart, p. 83.

[72]Ibid., p. 46; see also Moira A. Stewart, Ian R. McWhinney and Carol W. Buck, "The Doctor-Patient Relationship and Its Effect Upon Outcome" *Journal of the Royal College of General Practice* (in press).

[73]Ibid., p. 85.

[74]Ibid., pp. 135ff.

[75]Ludwig von Bertalanffy, *General Systems Theory* (New York: George Braziller, 1968).

[76]Willard Waller, *The Family: A Dynamic Interpretation* (New York: Dryden, 1938), p. 25.

[77]Irwin Savodnik, "Philosophy of Biology," in *Encyclopedia of Bioethics*, ed. Warren T. Reich (New York: Free Press, 1978), Vol. 1, pp. 127-32.

[78]William W. Meissner, "Theories of Personality," in *The Harvard Guide to Modern Psychiatry*, ed. Armand M. Nicholi, Jr. (Cambridge, Mass.: The Belknap Press, Harvard University Press, 1978), p. 129.

[79]Letha Scanzoni and John Scanzoni, *Men, Women and Change: A Sociology of Marriage and Family* (New York: McGraw-Hill, 1976), chap. 1.

[80]Ibid., p. 8.

[81]Walter Buckley, *Sociology and Modern Systems Theory* (Englewood Cliffs, N.J.: Prentice-Hall, 1967).

[82]Scanzoni and Scanzoni, p. 13.

[83]Janet Seely, "The Justification for Teaching About the Family System to Family Physicians," working paper at the W. K. Kellogg Centre for Advanced Studies in Primary Care, Montreal General Hospital.

[84]For example, the program for Kellogg Fellows at the W. K. Kellogg Centre for Advanced Studies in Primary Care at the Montreal General Hospital.

[85]Paul Ramsey, *The Patient as Person* (New Haven, Conn.: Yale University Press, 1970), p. 123.

[86]Theodore Lidz, *The Person* (New York: Basic Books, 1968), pp. xv-xix.

[87]Ibid., pp. xvi-xvii.

[88]Harold J. Cornacchia, David E. Smith and David J. Bentel, *Drugs in the Classroom*, 2nd ed. (St. Louis, Mo.: C. V. Mosby Co., 1978), p. 152.

[89]James E. Groves, "Taking Care of the Hateful Patient," *New England Journal of Medicine*, 298, No. 16 (20 April 1978), 883-87.

[90]Cf. D. O. Swann, "Health," in *The New Bible Dictionary*, ed. J. D. Douglas (Grand Rapids, Mich.: Eerdmans, 1962), p. 509.

[91]Johs. Pedersen, *Israel: Its Life and Culture* (London: Geoffrey Cumberlege,

1926), I & II, p. 311.

[92]Gerhard von Rad, "Shalom in the O.T.," in Gerhard Kittel, *Theological Dictionary of the New Testament,* trans. Geoffrey W. Bromiley (Grand Rapids, Mich.: Eerdmans, 1964), II, 402.

[93]Ps. 38:3; Is. 57:18-19; Jer. 6:14.

[94]J. Barton Payne, *The Theology of the Older Testament* (Grand Rapids, Mich.: Zondervan, 1962), p. 435.

[95]Ibid., p. 429.

Part IV

The Ministry of
Whole-Person Medicine

Chapter Eleven

The Ministry of Medicine in the Care of the Whole Person

Richard Sosnowski

What is the most painful and devastating question that can be asked about modern medical practice? It is not whether most doctors are up to date in their knowledge or in their techniques but whether too many of them know more about disease than about the person in whom the disease exists. . . .

The modern doctor strides forth into the world from medical school with a certificate of learning in one hand and a vast array of exotic medications and technological devices in the other. But the humans who look to him for help are as fragile and perplexed and vulnerable as they ever were. More than anything else, they want to know that they matter. They don't want anything to come between them and their doctors. . . . People want their doctors to be finely tuned human beings capable of exquisite tenderness, not impersonal and detached super-scientists. They want to feel that the physician who is examining them is thinking of nothing else. . . .

The physician celebrates computerized tomography. The patient celebrates the outstretched hand.[1]

Centuries ago, Plato said: "The great error in the treatment of the human body is that physicians are ignorant of the whole. For the part can never be well unless the whole is well."

Four hundred years later, Jesus of Nazareth, on one occasion of healing after another, indicated the relationship of spiritual integrity to physical health. He said, "Thy faith hath made thee whole" (Mt. 9:22; Mk. 5:34; 10:52; Lk. 17: 19 KJV).

In the nineteenth century, the biologically oriented psychology of Sigmund Freud reaffirmed the ancient principle that the mind and the body are interactive and interdependent. Thus it laid the groundwork for modern psychosomatic medicine. In 1938 Flanders Dunbar collected the widely scattered world literature in that field, and the following year the *Journal of Psychosomatic Medicine* began publication.

In the 1940s Paul Tournier of Switzerland began to put his concepts of medicine of the whole person into writing. He made a clear distinction between medicine of the whole person and psychosomatic medicine.

> Whole-person medicine goes rather beyond psychosomatic medicine while still being in full accord with it. . . . It implies a double view of man . . . that of the physical, chemical phenomena which determine and belong to the realm of the natural sciences, and that of his behavior as a person, as a spiritual being, free and responsible. . . . It is not sufficient to prescribe, to counsel, to exhort. It is necessary to understand profoundly the person of the patient. Man is not just a body and a mind. He is a spiritual being. It is impossible to know him if one disregards his deepest reality.

> Man—body, mind and spirit—is a unity. . . . Everyone understands what is meant by body, but I must make a clear distinction between mind and spirit. Mind, the psyche, is the domain of psychology: the intelligence, feeling, moral sense, etc. The spirit expresses itself through all these and also through the body, but it is neither the mind nor the body. It is concerned with the personal relationship of man with God.

In 1947 Dr. Tournier with Dr. Jean DeRouchemont of France and Dr. Maeder of Germany convened the Conference of Medicine de la Personne; such conferences have continued on an annual basis ever since. Those of us who have been privileged to attend them have been profoundly impressed.

One of the greatest impacts is the Bible study at the beginning of each scientific session—something unique in medical meetings. Dr. Tournier's admonition to his fellow physicians is this: "Study the Bible as clinicians, for there you will find the story of man's behavior."

Paul Tournier is now eighty. From his pen there still flow in beautiful proliferation his concepts and beliefs about the sacredness of the person. *The Healing of Persons, The Meaning of Persons, Person Reborn, The Adventure of Living, Guilt and Grace* and *A Place for You* are but a few of his books.

The Search for the Whole Person

How do you and I encounter the whole person? At the 1974 Conference of Medicine of the Whole Person in England, Dr. Bernard Harnik gave a diagrammatic description of what to look for. The circle was used because it represents wholeness. Most people encounter each other with reference to the superficial images listed in the circle. They communicate at that level and they relate to each other at that level. Most of the time no in-depth encounter is experienced and, therefore,

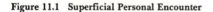

Figure 11.1 Superficial Personal Encounter

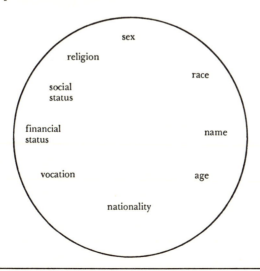

the level of true personhood is never reached. The real person of each participant in that kind of exchange remains hidden under multiple superficial images. The physician practicing medicine of the whole person attempts to see through all of those images to the real person at the center. If that is done from a Christian perspective another dimension is added: the physician searches for and tries to help the patient develop the image of Christ.

Now, lest this sound too evangelistic, let us remember that C. G. Jung—who surely did not become known for his Christian evangelism—considered Christ to represent the archetype of the self. Looked at psychologically, the figure of Christ as the symbol of the self acts like a magnet drawing disparate materials into their proper places. Christian theology proclaims reconciliation through Christ of our differences. In Jungian psychology, psychic wholeness is the attainment of true knowledge of the self. In Christian theology, spiritual wholeness comes through true knowledge of Christ, the psychological symbol of the self. It seems to me that Christian theology and Jungian psychology are close to saying the same thing: at the center of personhood there is psychologically the self; theologically, Christ.

One of the best ways to search for the whole person is to listen patiently and sensitively. How do we listen to the person of the individual? We listen for what the individual says verbally: the actual words. We listen also for what the individual says subverbally: the real meaning behind the words, the fear behind the bravado, the inadequacy behind the boasting, the hostility behind the sweetness. We listen and look for what the individual says nonverbally: in facial expression, tone of voice, body posture. This latter—some call it "body language"—can be seen in the forward, open posture; the rigid, defensive posture; the closed, remote posture; the fetal fist of insecurity; the slump of despair; the jutting chin of anger and aggression; the alcoholic breath at a morning appointment.

And what of the body language that we are broadcasting to the individual? Does it say that we are listening because we care or because we are trapped? The astrologer's position or the prolapsed-jawbone position or the Excedrin-headache position speak in loud nonverbal language to the individual. Touch is a powerful mode of communication. My willingness for my skin to be contiguous with your skin says eloquently that "I accept you."

When making hospital rounds, speeding in and out of patients' rooms or pacing the floor the entire time says, "I really don't have time for you." Standing quietly at the bedside or, better still, pulling up a chair for the same length of time as the pacer's visit, is a simple nonverbal communication that says convincingly, "You are worth my time." An impressive experiment was done with one group of patients and two groups of physicians. Both groups visited the patients for a timed two minutes. One group of physicians was instructed to pace around the room, not to touch the patient and not to make eye contact with the patient. The second group was instructed to stop at the bedside, touch the patient and make eye contact. When questioned, the patients all agreed that the first group visited no longer than two minutes at the most, but they thought that the second group had visited somewhere between five and ten minutes.

Colleagues have told me that it isn't fair to my other patients to spend so much time with any one of them. But the other patients haven't complained; they seem to know that if they should need it, I would spend the same amount of time with them. The urgency of his mission must have tempted Christ to hurry, hurry, hurry, but his mission was characterized by his complete giving of himself to each person in a calm and completely personal dialogue.

Tournier makes the point that medicine of the whole person begins with the person of the physician himself. In fact, in anticipation of this conference I told Dr. Tournier that I was being asked to present his viewpoint on the medicine of the whole person and asked what he would have me say. His reply was that he could not give me anything to say, because the way in which each physician implemented his views had to be decided and developed by the individual physician. Tournier sees the doctor and the patient each as, first of all, a person.

And he sees their relationship not as coldly objective and professional, but warmly and deeply interpersonal. He writes:

Practicing medicine in its technical aspect, we write prescriptions. They may be compared to the law of the Old Testament. In them we lay down what medicines the patient should take and the things he should do in order to get well. It is useful, but cold and impersonal. When we are aiming at practicing a whole medicine, a medicine of the person, which will help the patient to live, and awaken the forces of life within him, the important thing is no longer the prescription, but the personal bond between him and ourselves. We ourselves are involved.

These are, perhaps, startling words to some of us. They mean being ourselves as persons while ministering to our patients as persons. They do not mean sentimentality. They do not mean that we diminish our scientific acumen in arriving at a diagnosis or our therapeutic skill in treatment. But in addition to utilizing these faculties to the fullest extent, we also drop our masks which show just who we would like people to think we are. Our openness invites our patients nonverbally to drop their masks so that their real persons can be seen and heard. Then there is a therapeutic bond working both ways that cannot be measured in milligrams or cubic centimeters.

The Physician's Role

Let me make something clear: I am not advocating that we convert our roles into full-time counseling; I certainly have not done that and do not expect to. The fact simply is that, in our daily experience, deeply troubled and hurt people will come in, hoping we will either hear or see the real trauma in their lives. Either it will be the first time they have been able to bring themselves to speak of it to anyone, or else it represents a fairly desperate attempt—and perhaps the final one of many attempts—to have someone hear them.

Isn't it incumbent on us, then, as practitioners of the art of healing, to listen sufficiently to let the person know that he or she has been heard, to afford at least temporary stabilizing reassurance? After that, we can decide whether to see that person again for further discussion at a time more convenient to us, rather than right in the middle of our busy schedule (which is the time at which it usually happens initially) or whether to refer them to someone else. If psychiatric referral is decided on, semantics become important. "I'll have to send you to a psychiatrist." Negative response. "Let's ask the help of one more competent in this area." Positive response. You and I have remained with the person and not exiled him or sentenced her to the psychiatrist.

Two events early in my medical career probably started my thinking in the direction of the whole person. As I was entering medical school, my mother was diagnosed as having cancer. During the next two years, while she seemed to be losing that battle, I came to learn much more about the reaction of the *person* than I was to know for a long time about the disease—her apprehension, frustration, bewilderment and, yet, a resigned kind of courage. Even years later, when her malignancy was obviously arrested, I saw her translation of any new symptom into the ominous possibility of recurrence. It was a long time before I understood that much about the histopathology of malignancy.

Then, just as I graduated from medical school, my only brother was stricken with the most severe case of polio to survive that particular epidemic in our community. I came to understand what happens to the person of a powerful, robust, young man suddenly paralyzed from the waist down. I came to understand much more about those aspects than I understood for years about the neuropathology of poliomyelitis—the feeling of complete helplessness, the threatening uncertainty of what set of muscles was going to be paralyzed next and, yet, a stubborn optimism.

Those experiences and others have led me progressively to a commitment to medicine of the whole person. For many years my thoughts were not formulated into such clear terms as "medicine of the whole person." I simply realized with increasing conviction that patients' complaints and their real hurts were often far apart, and that if I listened I would hear the real hurt. I also realized that the real hurt frequently would have nothing to do with my practice of obstetrics and gynecology. What, then, was my responsibility?

That question led to another: Am I a physician who wants my patients to be healed, or am I a specialist who wants only a part of the patient to be healed?

Listening

If we listen, what will we hear? Here are some of the things I have heard.

I have heard the hollow laugh of a pretty young woman joking about the smallness of her breasts. When she returned from the examining room to my consultation room, I said, "You laughed and joked about your breast size a moment ago, but your laugh didn't sound real to me." Then she wept bitterly as she told me of her postpartum breast change—a very slight change really, but one which spelled diminished femininity to her. Making the whole situation worse was her husband's teasing. We spent time talking about the femininity of the *person* and putting into proper perspective the relationship of secondary sex characteristics to that femininity.

I have heard the greater-than-usual distress in the voice of a mother whose teen-age daughter I had diagnosed the day before as being pregnant. Medicine of the whole person quickly becomes medicine of the whole family. Don't they always sound distressed? Of course they do. But there was a more compelling note this time, so I went to their home. The father, a physician, had his right hand in a cast, having sustained a fracture the previous evening by banging the dining-room table in his desperateness and frustration. The mother and the father were on opposite sides of the room and the daughter in another corner. There was no communication at all. Often in such cases the unwed daughter is so filled with guilt and shame that she literally shuts herself off from her parents, thus denying herself the kind of support she longs for and needs, denying her parents the only avenue of compensation for their grief and frustration—to give her their love and loyalty. It is essential, then, that we bring child and parents back into communication with each other—not with indictment and defense, which is dual-logue, but through dialogue, which is accepting each other and hearing each other and responding rather than reacting. There is scarcely a time in the life of a family when it is more necessary for everybody to be on the same team, and you and I can coach them to that point. With this particular family, the coaching occupied the next two hours. When we said good-night, the three of them were standing in the doorway with their arms around each other.

I have heard the spiritual agony of a woman who between marriages had had an illegitimate pregnancy. When her only child, a son by the first marriage, was killed in Viet Nam, she considered it divine punishment for her unwed pregnancy. I found myself talking to her about God's forgiveness. Would a prescription for tranquilizers have solved her problem? I don't think so. Shouldn't she have sought help from pastor or priest? Perhaps. But she hadn't gone to him with the pregnancy, and she had come to me. My doing anything less than trying to meet her spiritual needs right then would have been to fail her.

In one week I have heard in the voices and seen in the faces of two patients domestic anguish masquerading as menopausal symptoms. Both were on hormonal therapy and both of them began their complaints by saying, "Your dose of estrogen is no longer adequate." Both women were suffering from nervousness, insomnia, crying and markedly increased hot flashes. It took only a few moments to test their estrogen levels and, in both cases, they were quite adequate. At that point I could have told them bluntly that they did not need any increase in estrogen dosage, or I could have simply written another prescription—this time for tranquilizers— but their distress made me ask what was happening to them in their personal lives.

The first patient had one son returning home from a broken marriage. Another son about to marry a girl with a malignant disease and a very compromised life expectancy. Understandably, her husband's stomach ulcer was bleeding. And, understandably, all of her menopausal symptoms were aggravated, and no amount of estrogen would have solved the problem. After listening to her articulate her stress burden, I simply talked with her about her life with her family. I tried to help her accept the limitations of her responsibility.

The second patient, who was an only child, had become completely incarcerated by the demands of her eighty-year-old mother. She had no life of her own, none with her husband, nor her children, nor her grandchildren. She had borne the burden to the breaking point. After hearing her out, I talked with her about the realities of one person's possessing another, about the limits of responsibility and about morally acceptable alternatives to her current situation. So far as I know, neither of those patients required any additional therapy.

I have heard the impatience and the anger of a terminal patient. Ministry to the dying requires our honesty and our time. One of the last meaningful services we can render is to be a patient's dependable source of information. If we lie, the patient will almost surely discover our deceit. The personal bond between physician and patient is then broken, and thereafter it is reduced to the technical relationship of prescriptions for narcotics.

Many of us in the medical profession find it difficult to accept death as an integral part of life. All of our teaching has been to save life and to restore health. Thus, the death of a patient spells personal professional defeat. Not wanting to be reminded of that, we tend to spend less and less time with the dying patient. The patient senses the decreasing frequency and duration of our visits and interprets that as personal worthlessness. Then, impending death becomes more humiliating and a hollow mockery of life.

I recall vividly a terminal patient who, in contrast to her usual uncomplaining serenity, became impatient and irritable. One evening she angrily demanded, "Are you not going to do anything for me?" Sitting down by the bedside and taking her hand, I simply recounted the events of her original exploratory surgery, the convalescence, the second surgery for obstruction and the current state of her condition. Then she said, "Thank you for telling me." The next morning, with her usual manner, she summoned her attorney and put her affairs in order. One week later, again during evening rounds, she asked, "Do you think it will be long now?" I answered that I hoped it would not, because now the only victory possible for her was to return to God. She said, "Don't make me wait," and I promised that my only medical efforts would be to keep her comfortable. That night she died quietly in her sleep.

Relating the events of one clinical situation will illustrate the significance of touch. One of our house staff called me in to talk to a woman having her six weeks' postpartum visit. She was covered from head to foot with the characteristic skin lesions of secondary syphilis. The resident physician had initiated the diagnostic procedures, but the patient was refusing to return to the clinic for either confirmation of the diagnosis or for treatment, although the vital importance of both had been explained. Her body language was one of total despair and dejection. I told her that I understood how devastating this news was and how it might threaten her marriage. I offered to help in that area. She continued to sit with head bowed, numb, mute. Then I discerned one small area on her bared shoulder that was free of lesions. Putting my hand there, I told her that I hoped she would do what she needed to do. Shortly after I left the examining room she promised the young physician that she would return the following day, and she did.

Medicine of the whole person is not a technique or a system or a methodology—but an attitude. It is an attitude at least partially characterized by an old quotation, "The duty of medicine is sometimes to heal; often to afford relief; and always to bring consolation."

How often you and I hear and see and sense that our patients living in this twentieth century are almost daily having to adapt to changing situations. If they cannot, they become lost in the whirlwind. They feel they have no place in the world.

Teilhard de Chardin was constantly caught in that dilemma of place. Should he follow his vocation as a priest or his vocation as a scientist? What was his place? In modern society the individuals, the families, who have no place are legion. Dr. Tournier's book *A Place for You,* speaks poignantly to this problem.

What extra dimension does the Christian physician have to offer in ministering to the whole person?

1. Sometimes we must help people work through their own self-judgment and guilt. They assume that their illness or injury represents divine punishment. Remember Jesus' explanation of the man who was blind from his birth: "Neither hath this man sinned, nor his parents: but that the works of God should be made manifest in him" (Jn. 9:3 KJV).

2. To minister to the whole person, we must to some extent feel the person's problems. In the Old Testament Isaiah speaks of one who "hath borne our griefs, and carried our sorrows" (Is. 53:4 KJV). He also gives us a good daily motto: "he hath sent me to bind up the brokenhearted" (Is. 61:1 KJV).

3. Increasingly patients are asking their physicians to talk to them about the meaning of life and death and about God. They are asking that we pray for them and with them. If we are so scientifically oriented that we dare not let our own spirituality show, we may deny our patients a great source of comfort and reassurance. If we fail to relate to the patient's spirituality, we may fail to utilize their greatest source of strength.

4. Finally, to minister to the whole person, especially to spiritual needs, there must be what I can only call a spiritual reaction between patient and physician. It may be such a powerful reaction that we feel emotionally and spiritually drained afterward. Yet we must be willing to take on some of our patients' hurts and to have some of our own spiritual strength transferred to them. Both Mark and Luke, in describing the healing of the woman with bleeding of twelve years' duration, spoke of Jesus' knowing that "virtue had gone out of him" at the moment of healing. There was a spiritual reaction between healer and healed.

For me, the experience of a spiritual reaction involving another person and myself has been my retrospective awareness of God's help. This has happened when I have been confronted suddenly with profound distress for which I was quite unprepared. Yet appropriate words were spoken and consolation was given. Looking back on the incidents, I have been certain that what was said and done did not originate with me. Surely it was God's responsive action to human need through me. Thus it was a spiritual reaction in which I was a participating instrument.

These, then, are some of the aspects of the ministry of medicine in the care of the whole person. Many of them are not new. But an exciting and relatively new realization is Dr. Tournier's thesis that as physicians seek to know and bring forth the real person in their patients, they find their own personhood enhanced toward wholeness.

Notes
[1]Editorial, *Saturday Review*, 22 July 1978.

Chapter Twelve

A Clinical View
of the Gospel

Bruce Larson

I have looked forward both to seeing Oral Roberts University for the first time and to interacting with men and women who represent an exciting and viable movement, not only in medicine but in human life.

A friend tells a wonderful story about a mother and her son. It seems that every Sunday morning this mother had a terrible time getting her son up to go to church. She shamed him, threw water in his face, pulled the covers off and did all kinds of ingenious things to get him up and going. One Sunday none of these tricks seemed to work. Finally, in a rage, the son got up stamping his foot. "Mother!" he shouted. "I will not go to church this Sunday! It is dull, boring and irrelevant. You can't give me a good reason why I should go." She said, "As a matter of fact, I can give you two good reasons why you should go" (mothers are always up to that sort of challenge). She said, "First of all, you are forty-four years old. Second, you are the minister."

Perhaps one of the reasons church can sometimes seem dull and boring is that we in the church act as if we were in the entertainment business. We think we must provide interesting sermons, beautiful music, exciting drama or whatever it is we do to entertain. We need to change our focus and realize instead that we are in the business of being channels of God for the healing and wholeness of people. There is nothing boring about that.

Let's think of a counterpart in the medical world. Suppose you doctors spent your days simply going to lectures on health, reading papers on health and holding meetings where great numbers gathered and talked about health, but you never treated a sick person. It would be the dullest job in the world. Somehow we have to become a community of faith together, doctors and lay people alike, pooling our resources. The church could be a place where God is back in the business of making people whole as the community of faith learns and works together.

Wholeness

I want to suggest two things that we Christian laypersons have learned from those of you in the medical community. The first is a new understanding of illness, of what it means to be sick. The second is an understanding of health as *wholeness*.

Some people at the beginning of our century have been God's pioneers in this new understanding. They have been like the mountain men who opened up the West, the first ones to go into unexplored forests and mountains to find out what was there. They notched the trees so that the rest of us could follow their trail and begin where they left off. In discovering what it means to be human beings from God's perspective, we thank God for a mountain man like Sigmund Freud, who showed that illness was more than just organic.

Other early pioneers in our century were people like Franz Alexander and Flanders Dunbar. They explored the whole psychosomatic field and talked about the emotional reasons for all kinds of illness. Their theories explored the relationship of illness to personality constellations.

William Osler, the father of North American medicine, was another such pioneer. That great medical man suggested to us that many patients get well because they have faith in the doctor's faith in the cure. So when a doctor loses faith in a certain procedure, whether it is surgery, drugs or physical therapy, that treatment becomes ineffective.

A pioneer like Paul Tournier has been helping us understand our personhood as over against the person in the mask or the personage. He is the father of one whole dimension of whole-person medicine.

Another mountain man notching trees was Hans Selye, who said that your health and longevity depend on how you handle stress (and you can't be alive and avoid stress) determines how whole and how healthy you are, how soon you will die and how well you will be during your life.

A more recent pioneer is James Lynch out of Johns Hopkins, who claims that loneliness is the number-one killer in America today and has statistics to prove it. According to Lynch, people who have become demonstratively lonely through death or divorce or any other circumstance become ill and die sooner. All of these pioneers have underscored the correlation between our health and our ability to relate to people in meaningful ways.

Actually our lifestyle is making a lot of us sick. A generation ago a town near Scranton, Pennsylvania, named Roseto was the subject of medical research because its citizens had almost no incidence of heart attack. Nobody under fifty had had a heart attack and in the over-fifty group they suffered only one-fourth the national average. The people were almost all first-generation Italian immigrants who worked in the mines in that area. They ate enormous quantities of pasta, lasagne, spaghetti, red wines and all sorts of rich things. Yet nobody got heart attacks.

Now, a generation later, that same town has four times the national heart-attack rate. They are now eating sensibly like Americans. Instead of pasta, they eat diet foods, skimmed milk and margarine. But their lifestyle has changed. They no longer have a sense of community. The residents commute long distances for better and higher paying jobs. Many of them are deeply in debt. They are competitive. They live like Americans.

The whole health-food thing is so interesting. I don't mean to offend you if you are a health-food person, but I'm not convinced that what you eat is going to make you what you are. To a degree that may be true, but Jesus said two thousand years ago to people who were *so careful* about what to eat, how to eat it, even about eating it from certain dishes, "Listen, it's not what goes into your mouth that kills you, it's what comes out of your mouth that kills you." I think that is just as true today. Right attitudes, right relationships are more important than right diet.

Understanding Health

We are grateful for the insight you in the medical profession are giving us about the meaning of illness. But beyond that and perhaps even more important, you are giving us a new understanding of health. The preamble to the World Health Organization says that "Health is more than the absence of illness." In other words, in theory, you could take away every sign of pathology in a patient and that person still might not be well. Health is more than not being sick. Health is wholeness.

A correlation for those of us in the church is that righteousness is more than the absence of sin. In theory, if you could be sinless, you still might not be righteous. You could be comatose in the hospital, being fed intravenously, incapable of sinning, but that doesn't make you a saint. That is not what we are talking about when we speak of righteousness.

Martin Luther was perhaps on the right track when he said, "Love God and sin boldly." You can squander your spiritual inheritance on not being bad and blow the whole thing. If you are going to live in the real world, trying to live out your Lord's command to love people as he has loved you, you will be deeply involved with people and you will occasionally sin against them by manipulation, withholding, insensitivity and just plain self-centeredness. There is no way, being who we are, that we can begin to love people and not sin occasionally or even frequently. Luther's statement to love God and sin boldly is definitely not a call to license. It means that when you sin, you should admit it, make restitution, confess, believe you are forgiven and move on to the business of loving and doing the positive thing.

We have overemphasized pathology. Tolstoy once said that all sick families are sick in their own way, but all healthy families look alike. If that's true, then to emphasize only the study of pathology is not very helpful. Even if you've studied the pathology of one sick person in detail, the next patient will be an entirely different person even if he or she has the same symptoms. But if you could find the plus, the self-actualizing agent (in Maslow's term), the reasons for health or wholeness in a patient, you have found something universal.

Understanding the Gospel

I want to say that the Bible is our greatest resource for helping people wholistically. The Bible is not a theological book. It is a record of God's interaction with humanity beginning with the Old Testament and throughout our Lord's own life and the lives of the early apostles. It is a remarkable record. The Bible is more than a book to be preached from or discussed, to be carried carefully to Sunday school or to use as a basis for our devotions. As long as we see the Bible as basically theological rather than practical we are going to miss the whole point of it.

We have to get a new mind-set in order to understand that the Bible was never meant to be a book of theology. We have distilled our theology from the events recorded in the Bible, but the Bible is a book about human behavior from God's point of view. It is a book about how life caves in if we disobey or ignore his will, or how life opens up if we will do and be faithful people. God had a purpose when he chose the people through whom he could make his ultimate revelation. They were to be a receptacle not just for stone tablets and laws but for the Incarnation itself. He chose a people whose language was not in the least philosophical. The Hebrew language is primarily verbs; it is action centered. When the gospel spread to the Greeks, the biblical events were interpreted through a new language, a much more philosophical language. But originally God revealed himself to a people of action and through a verb-centered language. The Bible is a clinical book

—a book about the interaction of God and Jesus Christ and the Holy Spirit with you and me as people.

It seems to me, as I read the Gospels, that Jesus was less concerned about healing the sick than about making people whole. He did not set out to hold all-day clinics. Rather he was busy living something out with a handful of disciples, traveling about, preaching and teaching, interacting with and challenging the authority figures. In the midst of those activities, people would interrupt him, bringing their sick to be healed. His focus was not on making the sick well but on bringing a new kind of life to all people, sick or well.

In the tenth chapter of John's Gospel, Jesus said, "I came that you might have life, and have it abundantly." The Greek words here convey the idea of life running over, coming out at the seams. That is why Jesus came. This is the basis of my belief that wholistic medicine grows out of the Christian faith. Jesus did not come to make us religious or even to make us good. He came that we might have life, pressed down, running over. The New Testament tells us that all of creation is standing on tiptoes to see the sons and daughters of God coming into their own. You may think that describes some sinless state, but according to Scripture there are already tens of billions of angels all over creation who are sinless. Angels are simply messengers of God, sent to do his will. But you and I are capable of a quality of life a sinless angel is not capable of —a kind of life that represents what it means to be a whole person.

Certainly we cannot ignore sickness. People break bones. They experience organ malfunctions. But only ten per cent of the sick people you doctors treat have broken bones, injuries, disease, in other words a treatable illness. But doctors cannot treat the great malaise of our time which is related to the search for life.

I want to suggest that if we take a clinical approach to some of the truths about life that we find in the gospel they can help us toward health and wholeness in our lives and in the lives of others. I want to discuss seven such specific truths, but of course one could list many more than that.

Accountability

The first truth is in the area of accountability and comes from Jesus' saying, "Where two or three are gathered together in my name, there am I in the midst of them." Does that mean that the Lord of creation, the Savior of the world, is somehow physically or spiritually more present with three people than with one? I don't believe it means that at all. Jesus meant that, for wholeness, we need accountability. When you are alone, you can deceive yourself. You will always lie to yourself. You will make wrong choices. You need to find some people to whom you can be accountable, who know you, who will pray with you, who will tell you the truth about yourself and hold you to your best.

This kind of accountability is the genius of Alcoholics Anonymous and of the Wesleyan class meetings. When people are accountable to each other in such a group, life bubbles up, and pathology is dealt with along the way. Week by week I can recount my self-defeating behavior, and the group can say, "Oh, Larson, get off that stuff." And I hear the rebuke and I can move on and find a more excellent way to deal with my wife, my children, my best friend or my worst enemy. The behavioral scientists know this. They say simply, "Behavior that is observed, changes." Sometimes your patients get well for that reason. They can tell you how much they are eating, whether or not their sex life is satisfactory, how often they go to church and if they are paying their bills. Once a week or once a month, they are accountable and that is therapeutic. The problem is, you haven't time to see most of your patients on that basis.

Culpability

We find a second life-truth that leads to wholeness in 1 John 1:9. "If we confess our sins, he is faithful and just, and will forgive our sins and cleanse us from all unrighteousness." I think that suggests that if we are to be whole people we need to acknowledge our culpability. We preachers have got to stop implying that if you are born again and Spirit-filled, you begin a life of innocence. Innocence is not a possibility. The gift God gives us by his grace is responsible guilt. When we can be responsibly guilty, we are on the way to health and wholeness. That is the best we are capable of. Only angels are perfect. We are not perfect and when we are wrong we need to say so.

The Bible gives us some classic examples of handling guilt. One is in the story of Aaron, Moses' brother. You know, God never chose Aaron as his messenger. Moses chose him. He said, "I can't do it alone, God, I stutter. But Aaron has been to seminary. He can preach!" Aaron was Moses' choice, and he proved to be a problem. While they were in the wilderness Moses went up on the mountain to receive the Ten Commandments and left Aaron in charge. When he didn't return immediately, the Israelites got panicky. Certain that Moses had left permanently, they said, "Let's go back to the familiar ways of Egypt. Let's build some idols and have a party." Moses returned to find them worshiping a golden calf and holding an orgy. So Moses angrily confronted Aaron. "Aaron, what in thunder have you done? You've built a golden calf and you have God's people worshiping Baal." Aaron's reply in something of a free translation, was "Moses, do you think I would build a golden calf? You see, we missed you. We threw a party, had a bit too much to drink and got carried away. We threw our rings and jewelry in the fire and the first thing you know, out came a golden calf."

It's like the answer that Cain, the first murderer, gave to God in the book of Genesis. God asked, "Where is your brother?" If only Cain could have said, "I killed him, Lord. I couldn't stand that son-of-a-gun. You always loved him more than me." If he had said that, reconciliation would have been possible. Instead he pretended innocence. He said, "How do I know? Am I my brother's keeper?" You see, the key to receiving grace is to acknowledge you are your brother's murderer by your indifference, your carelessness. All of us are responsible for withholding, for sins of omission and commission. When we can take responsibility for our guilt, the floodgates of heaven will open.

A friend of mine runs a Christian halfway house. It is a place to go if you aren't quite ready for padded walls but you can't take it at home anymore. You can go there for a few weeks and sort out your life and pray. But there is a sign up over the fireplace that says, "Do you want to be right or well? You can't be both." My friend says, "Most of the people who come here believe they are victims of the terrible things people have done to them over the years. And when they can stop justifying themselves, stop listing all the ways in which they have been wronged, stop having to prove they are really right in every situation, they can begin to get well." For those people, responsible guilt is the first step toward healing.

Someone once said, "To sin is man's condition. To pretend that he is not a sinner, that is man's sin." And you and I as healers, medical or theological, have got to love people to the place where they can say, "I blew it." We can say, "Friend, join the human race."

Responsibility

A third life-truth is found in the story of the man healed by the pool of Bethesda. It concerns the whole matter of taking responsibility for your life. The man had been lying there crippled for thirty-eight years, yet Jesus said, "Wilt thou be made whole?" ("Do you want to be healed?" is the modern translation.) Perhaps Jesus was suggesting that some of us prefer being professionally sick. We get preferential treatment at home. When we develop a migraine, people defer to us. When we choose to be well, we don't get preferential treatment. We've got to go back to work and take on our share of the daily chores and live like normal people. Jesus was asking the man by the pool if he was willing to take that kind of responsibility for his life. The invalid's reply was far from a straightforward yes. He said, "These people who are supposed to put me into the pool never get me there at the right time." In other words, "I am in this condition because other people have failed me."

Jesus performed many kinds of miracles. The raising of Lazarus, for example, is a real mind blower. Lazarus had been dead three days, yet Jesus said, "Come forth." That's one kind of miracle—the healing of the hopeless case, someone so far gone he or she cannot possibly cooperate in the cure. But another kind of miracle may occur because you decide to take responsibility for your own health. God may be saying, "Have you had enough? Are you tired of being in this state? I'm reminded of a cartoon I once saw. Two frogs are sitting on a lily pad and one said to the other, "You know, I tried that prince bit for a while, but frankly I missed eating flies." Healing may come when we can say to each other, "Hey, have you had enough flies today? If not, eat some more. Eat them until you're tired of flies and want to be a prince or princess."

I think the whole point of the story of the man by the pool is that people must take responsibility for their own lives. We can't make that choice for somebody else, and Jesus can't make it for us. We're told that the hardness of God is kinder than the softness of man. Instead of giving sympathy to somebody who is evading responsibility, we can hold out hope and say, "Hey, I think you can change."

So far I've been saying that as we read the Bible clinically, we find we are urged to be accountable, culpable and responsible, and all three of those attitudes are part of being a whole person. I'd like to add three more attributes to those, the three found in 1 Corinthians 13: faith, hope and love.

Faith

Faith is not just something we preach about emotionally in order to get people to come forward and make a decision, though that's certainly valid. After we have come forward to the altar by faith and given our life to Jesus, faith requires that we choose to lose our lives for his sake day by day. The clinical word for faith is *risk*. Because you believe in Jesus you say, "I'm going to risk my money, my reputation, my time, my energies. I'm going to bet on people and causes though I may never get any rewards. I may be rejected or even laughed at but I'm going to begin to live a life of risk."

When I turned forty-five I went to my doctor for a checkup and he said, "Well, you're in pretty good shape. But I'll tell you what you've got to do. When middle age hits, you've got to begin to fight the inclination toward security and a safe life.

That's what old age is all about, the inability to take any more chances. I hit forty-five a couple of years ago and I took up flying. I fly two hours a week and it's scary. But I think I'm a better doctor and a better husband and a better Christian because I choose risk for those two hours a week."

I couldn't afford a plane, but I immediately went out and bought a motorcycle and I rode it to my office each day. And, believe me, that was risky. But I think I understand what my doctor was saying about the need to reverse the usual trend to become safer, more conservative theologically and politically, more secure financially, more stable and safe professionally. But risk for risk's sake is not particularly productive. We need to move on to creative risk taking for God and his causes, and that's what faith is all about.

Hope

Just as essential to wholeness is hope. Hope is a sense of your destiny that is not based on your track record. You and I can help each other with this. You cannot plot your future from your past history, your school record, your marriage and your employment record. It is not confined to some neat graph that predicts where you are going on the basis of where you've been. The futurologists tell us they were wrong twenty years ago predicting the population growth, oil production or world food supplies on that basis. They say, "We thought we could predict the future on the basis of the past with our bell-shaped curves and straight lines. Now we know that the future is systemic and not linear for humankind, for nations, for churches, for families and for individuals."

Your future is *not* predetermined by past performance. God gave us the gift of choice. People with a whole record of failure can have a whole new series of choices today that can change the course of their lives. This is what hope is all about, the belief that something good is going to happen, and this kind of hope is a gift of God.

Years ago when I was studying psychology at Boston University I read about some tests done on rats. They put identical litters in two identical vats of water to see how long they could stay afloat. One vat was placed in a dark room with no visual stimulation and those rats drowned in an average of thirty-seven minutes. The other rats were placed in a lighted room where they could see other live rats above them moving about and behaving normally. Those rats lasted forty hours. Given hope, those rats displayed unbelievable stamina.

Hope is not just some elusive feeling about the Second Coming (though I believe in the Second Coming). God says hope makes a difference in your life in the here and now. Whatever your track record physically, mentally, morally, spiritually, the future can be different. If you lose your job, if you retire, if your spouse leaves you, your best friend betrays you, it's not the end.

I'm an admirer of Maggie Kuhn, founder of the Gray Panthers. At seventy-plus she said, "Listen, I'm not old." And she organized a bunch of senior citizens who tried to change America. They've got hope and they're going to die young as late as possible.

Love

In addition to faith and hope, to be a whole person from a biblical or clinical perspective we need the gift of love. Jesus loved us and died for us and that is ultimate love. He tells us to "love as I have loved you." People who love stay well, they get well, they are whole people.

We tend to think our real problem is the people around us who grab our parking space, pressure us, nag us and don't love us enough. Yet we're told that the highest rates of suicide, alcoholism and drug addiction are found in the least populated states, like Montana. When you live alone, something destructive takes place. Oddly enough, those problems are not nearly so acute in the ghettos and the overpopulated cities.

The way into a loving and intimate relationship is through vulnerability, through opening up to other people. The Scripture says, "How can you love God whom you have not seen if you cannot love your neighbor whom you have seen?" If you really love God, is there one person who knows all about you, whom you trust and whom you care for—whom you love?

Joy

Finally, health and wholeness are synonymous with the gift of joy. Jesus said, "I came that you might have joy. That my joy might be in you, that your joy might be full." God's saints are often hilarious people. God tells us we are to have joy. But it takes great courage to be happy. It takes the grace of God for you or me to choose to be happy, fulfilled people. You can't begin to lose your life if you haven't got a worthwhile life to lose. There is nothing Christian about being grim.

Joy has healing properties. Norman Cousins, editor of the *Saturday Review of Literature,* was healed some years ago. The doctors told him he had one chance in five hundred. He said, "Doctor, if that's the case, I'd like your permission to take over my own care." The doctor agreed. Cousins said, "First, I'm going to move out of the hospital. It will save me a ton of money and it's more germ-free and more fun." So he moved to a hotel room and began a course of self-treatment. He got his relationships straightened out and began to love people. But beyond that, he believed that humor is therapeutic. He rented old Marx Brothers and Laurel and Hardy films. A friend sent him old "Candid Camera" reruns. Every day he watched some of those films. After an afternoon of belly laughs he found his vital signs were up. Eventually, he experienced a total cure, and laughter was a big part of that cure.

I'm suggesting that a lot of people are sick because of joylessness, and you can remedy that. I believe we are in a great time in the church and that those of you in the medical profession can be pivotal prophetic thinkers for that time. But to practice the medicine of the whole person you're going to need all the help you can get from the lay people of the Christian church. Together we could begin to practice the healing ministry of the first-century church. The fifth chapter of Acts describes the church as it met on Solomon's porch. There was no official healing service but the sick and afflicted gathered there, and they got well around those early Christians. The entire body of Christ as represented by that early church was a healing force, and I believe we can be that today. That is the challenge of wholistic medicine.

Contributors

David F. Allen is assistant professor of psychiatry in the School of Medicine at Yale University. He was born in the Bahamas and received his medical education at the University of St. Andrews in Scotland and Guy's Hospital in London. He took his residency at Boston City Hospital and was a Kennedy Foundation Fellow in Medical Ethics at Harvard School of Public Health. With his wife, Vickie, Dr. Allen has recently written a book entitled *Ethical Issues in Mental Retardation: Tragic Choices, Living Hope* (1979).

Lewis Penhall Bird (S.T.M., Ph.D.) is the eastern regional director of the Christian Medical Society (Havertown, Pa.). He is also a member of the associate faculty of the Kellogg Centre for Advanced Studies in Primary Care of McGill University. He has served as a consultant to The Joseph P. Kennedy, Jr. Foundation project on adolescent pregnancy and is the author of *The Ten Commandments in Modern Medicine* (1965) and coauthor of *Learning to Love* (1971). He has also contributed articles to the *Dictionary of Christian Ethics, Is It Moral to Modify Man?* and *Horizons of Science.*

John R. Brobeck is Herbert C. Rorer professor of medical sciences at the University of Pennsylvania School of Medicine. He was born in Colorado and educated at Wheaton College, Northwestern University (Ph.D.) and Yale University (M.D.). He was a faculty member at the Yale University School of Medicine for ten years and chairman of the department of physiology at the University of Pennsylvania School of Medicine for eighteen years. His research interests include physiological control systems, temperature regulation, energy balance and food intake.

Arthur J. Dyck is Mary B. Saltonstall professor of population ethics at Harvard School of Public Health and a member of the faculty of Harvard Divinity School. He was born in Saskatoon, Saskatchewan, is married and has two children. He was educated at Tabor College, the University of Kansas (M.A.) and Harvard University (Ph.D.) and has authored numerous scholarly articles and two books: *On Human Care: An Introduction to Ethics* (1977) and *Ethics in Medicine* (coeditor, 1977).

Robert L. Herrmann is professor and chairman of biochemistry in the School of Medicine and Dentistry at Oral Roberts University. In the past he has served as associate dean for biomedical sciences at ORU and for seventeen years as a faculty member at Boston University School of Medicine. He attended Purdue University (B.S.) and Michigan State (Ph.D.) and was a Damon Runyon Fellow at the Massachusetts Institute of Technology. He presently serves on the boards of the Christian Medical Society and the American Scientific Affiliation.

James F. Jekel (M.D., M.P.H.) is associate professor of public health at Yale Medical School, where he has taught since 1967. His research interests include the problems of adolescent pregnancy, evaluation of health programs and the implications of religious faith for health-care delivery, particularly prevention. He lives in Hamden, Connecticut, with his wife and four children and is an elder in the Westminster Presbyterian Church.

Bruce Larson is a Presbyterian minister with a graduate degree in psychology from Boston University. A former president of Faith at Work, he is presently the director of the Group Research and Individual Learning Project and a visiting Fellow at Princeton Theological Seminary. He and his wife, Hazel, who is an editor, live on Sanibel Island. His many books, which have sold over two million copies, include these titles: *Dare to Live Now* (1965), *Living on the Growing Edge* (1968), *No Longer Strangers* (1971), *The Relational Revolution* (1976) and *The Meaning and the Mystery of Being Human* (1978).

Balfour Mount is professor of surgery at McGill University and director of the Palliative Care Service at the Royal Victoria Hospital, the first comprehensive university-based hospital service for terminal care and bereavement follow-up. He was educated at Queen's University, did postgraduate work at McGill University and undertook fellowships at the Royal College of Surgeons (Canada), Memorial Sloan Kettering Cancer Center and Jackson Research Laboratories (Bar Harbor, Me.). In 1979 he was awarded the Queen's Silver Jubilee Medal.

Robert M. Nelson is completing studies in medicine and theology at Yale University. His primary interests include pediatrics and biomedical ethics. He has been actively involved in the International Conference of Christian Medical Students and is a candidate for ordination in the Reformed Church of America.

Edmund D. Pellegrino is president of The Catholic University of America, professor of philosophy and biology at The Catholic University and professor of clinical medicine at Georgetown University. He was educated at St. John's University and New York University (M.D.) and has received numerous honorary degrees. He has authored many scholarly articles and the book *Humanism and the Physician* (1979). He has previously served on the faculty of Yale University and the State University of New York at Stony Brook and as a professor and vice president for health affairs in the University of Tennessee System.

J. Richard Sosnowski (B.S., M.D., FACOG, Diplomate of the American Board of Obstetrics and Gynecology) is associate dean of the College of Medicine and professor of obstetrics and gynecology of the Medical University of South Carolina. He is the author of numerous scholarly articles and the cofounder of the steering committee of Medicine and Ministry of the Whole Person Conference in America. He is also a licensed Episcopal lay reader and chalicer at St. Michael's Church in Charleston, S.C.

Granger E. Westberg is president and director of Wholistic Health Centers, Inc., and clinical professor of preventive medicine at the University of Illinois at the Medical Center, Chicago. A native of Chicago, he was educated at Lutheran School of Theology and the University of Chicago. He has spent many years as a parish pastor, hospital chaplain and member of medical school faculties. He is the author of several books including *Nurse, Pastor and Patient, Good Grief* and *Community Psychiatry and the Clergyman*.